Anti-Inflammatory Cookbook for Beginners

Easy and Healthy Recipes to Reduce Inflammation and Boost Autoimmunity. Including a 28-day Meal Plan and 10 Simple Physical Exercises for Everyone

Rosa Baker

Table of Contents

Introduction

Anti-inflammatory medication is the answer if your joints, muscles, or tendons hurt when you move. Whether it's taking corticosteroids (as prescribed by your doctor), using an over-the-counter cold remedy containing ibuprofen, or adopting a healthier diet, such as substituting fresh fruit and vegetables for processed foods. Anti-inflammatories are becoming more common as people become more active to combat conditions like osteoarthritis and carpal tunnel syndrome. However, some doctors prescribe them for headaches caused by ongoing migraines that are exacerbated by physical activity.

To control inflammation, eat more anti-inflammatory foods and fewer inflammatory foods. You should try to eat a wide variety of foods that are high in nutrients, healthy fats, and antioxidants. In a nutshell, this is the anti-inflammatory diet concept.

There are foods that cause inflammation, and foods that help reduce it. Processed foods, foods with added sugar, red meats, and alcohol are discouraged or limited in the anti-inflammatory diet. Instead, it favors fruits and vegetables, omega-3 fatty acid-rich foods, whole grains, lean protein, healthy fats, and spices. These anti-inflammatory foods provide a lot of antioxidants, which are important because they help the body get rid of free radicals. Our bodies naturally produce antioxidants to help remove free radicals; however, they occasionally require assistance from dietary antioxidants as well. Although free radicals are a byproduct of certain processes such as metabolism, their levels in the body can be increased by external irritants such as stress or poor diet.

Once you have completed reading, I invite you to leave a review on this book. This would mean so much to me as it would help the dissemination of this material; you know I have been working hard on this product, and I really hope you enjoy it!

Chapter 1. Benefits of an Anti-Inflammatory Diet

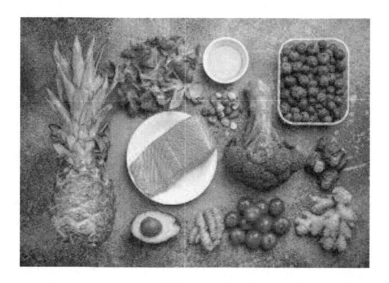

Principles of the Anti-inflammatory Diet

Consume less sugar: This is crucial to keep in mind. When I say "sugar," I don't just mean table sugar. Once in the body, refined carbohydrates are converted to sugar. White bread, white rice, and French fries are examples of refined carbohydrates. According to the American Heart Association (2018), men should consume approximately 9 tsp of sugar per day, while women should consume approximately 6 tsp. I know chocolate and cookies are tempting, but we must resist and reach for some fruit instead.

Consume less dairy: While fermented dairy products, such as yogurt, are safe to consume, fresh dairy products can occasionally cause inflammation.

Consume plenty of fresh fruits and vegetables: These are excellent sources of antioxidants as well as vitamins and fiber.

Consume omega-3-rich foods such as: This fatty acid is frequently deficient in our diet. We get a lot of Omega-6 because it's in vegetable oils and processed foods, but it needs to be balanced out with Omega-3.

Avoid processed foods: The anti-inflammatory diet emphasizes fresh and wholesome foods. I believe we can all agree that processed foods are bad for our bodies. Meal planning will greatly assist you in avoiding these foods.

The diet is all about filling up your meals with all those food items that can fight against inflammation. Also, you will have to cut out all those food items that tend to contribute to inflammation. The anti-inflammatory diet is more like a lifestyle than any traditional diet. It is an eating plan that helps in minimizing or reducing low-grade inflammation within your body. Ideally, you will have to increase your consumption of veggies and fruits every day, limit your consumption of dairy and red meat, opt for complex carbs, and stay away from processed food items. You will also have to consume foods that are filled with omega 3, such as anchovies, salmon, mussels, and halibut.

The Plan to Get the Best From Your Anti-Inflammatory Diet

1. Fiber must be an important component of your anti-inflammatory diet plan.

Fiber aids in the health of your gut. Dietary fiber is also important for maintaining healthy blood glucose levels. Fiber also improves insulin sensitivity in the body.

2. Your nutrient supplements are fruits and vegetables.

Those looking for the best nutrient supplements have every reason to give up their search. Fruits and vegetables provide the majority of the nutrients needed for a healthy body and mind. They're loaded with vitamins, minerals, and antioxidants. They are easy to digest and aid in the reduction of inflammation.

You must consume at least 4–5 servings of fruits and vegetables per day. Anti-inflammatory foods include leafy greens, cruciferous vegetables, and fruits. If you leave them out, your anti-inflammatory diet will be inefficient and ineffective. They add flavor to your life and make you look as healthy and energetic as they do.

3. Crucifers, in conjunction with onion, ginger, and garlic, can work wonders for your health.

It's no secret that cruciferous vegetables like broccoli, cauliflower, and Brussels sprouts are high in nutrients. Their anti-inflammatory properties are extremely potent. You can boost their potency and flavor by adding ginger, garlic, and onion to your recipes. They work together to strengthen your immune system. Adding onion, ginger, and garlic to your dishes will also add flavor. You can also experiment with other spices for flavor.

4. Consuming more than 10% saturated fat can be detrimental.

Saturated fats can be harmful to your health. They can raise the risk of heart disease and cause free radicals to be released. You should not consume more than 20 grams of saturated fat per 2000 calories per day.

Red meat consumption must be reduced. It is difficult to digest and is high in fat. Marinate it with herbs, spices, vinegar, and fresh fruit juices before eating it to reduce the buildup of toxic compounds during cooking.

5. Omega-3 fatty acids are crucial.

Omega-3 fatty acids are abundant in fruits, vegetables, seafood, and nuts. You must consume a sufficient amount of those foods on a daily basis. Omega-3 fatty acids are critical for reducing inflammation and lowering the risk of chronic inflammation-related diseases. Cancer, arthritis, heart disease, and neurodegenerative disorders are just a few of the diseases that can be avoided by eating omega-3 fatty acids.

6. Increase your consumption of cold water fish.

Wild cold water fish such as salmon, mackerel, and trout are high in omega-3 fatty acids. They also contain the majority of the other necessary vitamins and minerals. Eating wild caught cold water fish on a daily or weekly basis will significantly boost your immunity. These fish contain all of the antioxidants required as part of an anti-inflammatory diet. If you do not want to eat fish or have difficulty obtaining wild-caught cold water fish, you can take molecularly distilled fish oil supplements instead. It would be extremely unfortunate to miss out on either of the options.

7. For the best results, use healthy oils.

Food may not appear complete without oils and fat, but being careless with your oil selection can cost you a lot of money. Bad oil can harm your heart and promote the production of free radicals. Although your body requires fat, it does not have to be bad fat.

There are numerous healthy alternatives to oils, such as virgin and extra virgin olive oil. You can also use canola or sunflower oil that has been expeller pressed. These are high in polyphenols, which act as antioxidants.

8. Use fruits and spices to enhance the flavor of your meals.

It is critical to understand that if you do not exercise self-control, all your hard work and self-control will be for naught. Taste is an important aspect of life, and without it, things can become monotonous. Looking for it in refined sugar and artificial sweeteners, on the other hand, can be a big mistake. These products not only cause an excess of fructose accumulation, but they may also cause insulin resistance and increase the risk of type 2 diabetes.

Fruits are natural sugar substitutes. The sugar content of the fruits will aid in blood sugar regulation, and the digestive fiber will absorb any excess glucose. Fruits can add flavor to your meals while also improving your health. Spices are another way to add flavor to dishes.

9. 1 or 2 servings of beans and legumes per day will get you a long way.

Most vegetables lose nutrients when they are overcooked. Beans and legumes, on the other hand, do not fall into this category. They are versatile and provide essential minerals, protein, and soluble fiber. They are both tasty and nutritious. Leaving them out of your daily anti-inflammatory diet will result in a deficiency.

10. Physical activity is also essential.

A very important fact that you must never forget is the importance of physical activity in your anti-inflammatory diet. Physical activity stimulates your immune system and helps your body in fighting inflammation. Your system can absorb the required nutrients fast and fight better for chronic illnesses. Even small amounts of physical activity, like a brisk walk, can help in regulating your hormones and maintain a healthy balance. You will feel more refreshed and rejuvenated.

The Importance of Anti-Inflammatory Diet

Choosing an anti-inflammatory diet is a good idea for our health. Anti-inflammatory foods are high in antioxidants and vitamins, which slow the inflammatory response.

An anti-inflammatory diet is not a new concept; it has been around for a while. Many people have tried it and had great success. You might be surprised to learn that your favorite cuisine can cause inflammation in your body.

Anti-inflammatory diet benefits heart health, according to a Northwestern University study, foods high in omega 3 fatty acids, such as fish, nuts, and plants, can help protect the cardiovascular system from inflammation. Eating fish twice a week can thus cut the risk of developing heart disease in half.

An anti-inflammatory diet will benefit your joints: Anti-inflammatory diets may reduce your risk of osteoporosis by protecting your joints. The explanation is that omega-3 fatty acids can help keep your bones healthy and strong. Furthermore, according to the National Osteoporosis Foundation, anti-inflammatory diets contain antioxidants that can aid in the fight against this condition.

An anti-inflammatory diet will benefit your gut: A common question is, "Why does my stomach hurt?" If you have irritable bowel syndrome (IBS) or pouchitis, foods high in fiber and anti-inflammatory chemicals, such as fruits, vegetables, and whole grains, may help relieve your discomfort.

Following an anti-inflammatory diet may help you avoid becoming obese. An anti-inflammatory diet warns against overeating, which can lead to fat tissue buildup and obesity.

Obesity and an inflammatory diet may be related in a variety of ways. Consuming more refined carbohydrates, processed meats, and junk food is one inflammatory diet. Because these meals are low in calories and fiber, a person will have to eat more to compensate for the calorie deficit and lack of satiety. Two, someone who consumes an inflammatory diet may spend more time indoors, encouraging them to consume more calories while moving less.

People who are already suffering from inflammatory disorders may benefit from an anti-inflammatory diet in particular. Anti-inflammatory diets, for example, that exclude refined sugars and carbohydrates, may result in type 2 diabetes, metabolic syndrome, and obesity. An anti-inflammatory diet instead suggests eating whole grains like brown rice, which is high in fiber and has a low glycemic index.

An anti-inflammatory diet may also aid in fatigue. The inflammation indicates that the immune system is functioning properly. When the immune system is completely dedicated, histamine levels rise, making a person sleepy, tired, and cranky. The immune system's activities are supposed to make you tired, allowing your body to slow down and conserve energy. Fatigue is also thought to promote rest and healing rather than limiting the body further. An anti-inflammatory diet helps to reduce or eliminate inflammation, which reduces or eliminates the fatigue-causing effects of the immune system.

An anti-inflammatory diet that has nothing to do with obesity may aid in weight loss. Even if you are not obese, you may be overweight or on the verge of becoming obese. The high consumption of refined carbs and sugars is blamed for unintentional weight gain and other non-dietary reasons, such as sedentary lifestyles. Refined carbohydrate foods are low in nutrients, requiring more calories than necessary to meet calorie requirements.

An anti-inflammatory diet may aid in your sleep. Diet may contribute to poor sleep quality or an inconsistent sleep pattern in a variety of ways. When you eat an inflammatory diet, you will have difficulty sleeping on a regular basis, and when you do, it will be of poor quality. An inflammatory diet can cause eating issues, such as waking up in the middle of the night to eat, which can disrupt the quality and length of sleep. Due to fatigue, you may require frequent episodes of brief sleeping, which will disrupt your night's sleep. Fortunately, an anti-inflammatory diet can help you sleep better by lowering inflammation and ensuring that your meals are calorie and mineral balanced.

The biggest benefit of following an anti-inflammatory diet is that it can help reduce your risk of heart disease. Studies have shown that people who follow an anti-inflammatory diet are significantly less likely to develop heart disease than those who don't. Why is this? Well, an anti-inflammatory diet helps reduce the inflammation in your body, which is linked with the development of heart disease.

The Foods to Eat

- Kale and spinach are examples of dark leafy greens.
- Blackberries, blueberries, and cherries
- Grapes
- Cauliflower and broccoli
- Grass tea
- Beans and lentils
- Coconut and avocado
- Olives
- Olive oil
- Nuts such as walnuts, almonds, pistachios, pine nuts, and others
- Salmon and sardines are examples of coldwater fish (and other kinds of fish as well)
- Cinnamon, turmeric, and other spices
- Chocolate
- Watermelon
- Eggs
- Tomatoes

Foods to Avoid

Red meat: Red meat is a major source of inflammation in the body. It is known to increase 3 blood markers associated with heart disease and cancer. Homocysteine, C-reactive protein (CRP), and lipoprotein are examples of these (a).

Trans fats are linked to an increased risk of heart disease, stroke, diabetes, and inflammatory diseases such as Crohn's and rheumatoid arthritis.

Whole milk: According to a study published in *Nutrition Research*, drinking whole milk can cause inflammation in overweight adults.

When exposed to sugar, the body can produce more inflammatory proteins. This increase has been linked to a variety of health problems, including asthma, rheumatoid arthritis, and Alzheimer's disease.

Blue #1 and #2 dyes are frequently used in food products to make them appear more vibrant and appealing. These synthetic colors have been linked to an increased risk of allergies, cancer, ADHD, and inflammation.

Expensive juices: Expensive juices, such as pomegranate juice, are expensive because these "superfoods" are so good for you that you have to pay more for them.

Caffeine is a natural stimulant that can increase energy levels, but it can also cause an increase in inflammation in the body.

Processed meats, such as bacon, sausage, and ham, are frequently high in sodium and preservatives, both of which are known to cause inflammation.

Processed foods, particularly fast food, are high in added salt, sugar, and other additives that cause a lot of inflammation in the body.

Chapter 2. Breakfast Recipes

1. Mexican Breakfast Toast

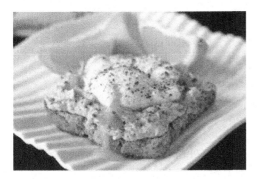

Preparation Time: 5 minutes

Cooking Time: 20 minutes

Servings: 2

Ingredients:

- 2 slices sprouted bread, toasted
- 2 tbsp hummus
- ½ cup spinach, chopped
- ¼ red onion, sliced
- ½ cup sprouts
- 1 avocado, thinly sliced
- ¼ tsp Himalayan salt

Spicy Yogurt

- 3 tbsp yogurt, unsweetened
- ½ lime, juiced
- 1 tsp cumin
- 1 tsp cayenne

Directions:

1. In a small bowl, prepare the Spicy Yogurt by combining all the Spicy Yogurt ingredients and whisking well to combine.
2. Place toast slices on plates and spread a tbsp of hummus on each. Place spinach on each slice, and then Spicy Yogurt, red onion, sprouts, and avocado. Sprinkle each with salt and serve.

Nutrition:

- Calories: 438 kcal
- Carbohydrates: 15 g
- Protein: 23 g
- Fat: 36 g
- Saturated Fat: 12 g
- Sodium: 1457 mg
- Fiber: 3 g

2. Italian Breakfast Hash

Preparation Time: 35 minutes

Cooking Time: 30 minutes

Servings: 2

Ingredients:

- 2 sweet potatoes, peeled and cubed into ½-inch pieces
- 2 tbsp olive oil
- ½ red onion, chopped
- ½ red bell pepper, halved and sliced
- ½ green bell pepper, halved and sliced
- 1 garlic clove, minced
- ½ tsp Himalayan salt
- ½ tsp black pepper, crushed
- ¼ tsp paprika
- 4 fresh sage leaves, thinly sliced
- 1 tsp oregano
- ¼ tsp red chili flakes
- 1 cup tempeh, crumbled
- 1 tbsp parsley, chopped

Directions:

1. Place sweet potato cubes in a medium pot over medium-high heat. Bring to a boil and let cook for 5 minutes. Potatoes should be tender, but not mushy. Drain and set aside.
2. Heat oil in a large skillet over medium-low heat. Add onion, bell peppers, garlic, and sweet potatoes. Cook for 10 minutes, stirring frequently.
3. Stir in the salt, pepper, paprika, sage, oregano, and chili flakes. Cook for 2 minutes, and then crumble in the tempeh. Cook another 2 minutes and then remove from heat.
4. Garnish with parsley before serving.

Nutrition:

- Calories: 43 kcal
- Carbohydrates: 4 g
- Protein: 1 g
- Fat: 3 g
- Sodium: 110 mg
- Fiber: 1 g
- Sugar: 1 g

3. Papaya Breakfast Boat

Preparation Time: 5 minutes

Cooking Time: 0 minutes

Servings: 2

Ingredients:

- 1 papaya, cut lengthwise in half, and seeds removed
- 1 cup yogurt, unsweetened
- 1 lime, zested
- 3 tbsp raw oats
- 1 tbsp coconut, unsweetened, shredded
- ½ banana, sliced
- ¼ cup raspberries
- 1 tbsp walnuts, chopped
- 1 tsp chia seeds
- 1 tsp raw honey

Directions:

1. Place papaya halves on plates and place yogurt on top of each.
2. Then top each half with lime zest, oats, coconut, banana, raspberries, walnuts, and chia seeds.
3. Drizzle with honey and serve.

Nutrition:

- Calories: 60 kcal
- Carbohydrates: 5 g
- Protein: 6 g
- Fat: 3 g
- Sodium: 90 mg
- Fiber: 1 g
- Sugar: 1 g

4. Summer Medley Parfait

Preparation Time: 10 minutes

Cooking Time: 0 minutes

Servings: 2

Ingredients:

- ⅓ cup raw cashews
- ½ tbsp raw honey
- ½ tsp vanilla extract
- ¼ tsp almond extract
- 1 tsp lemon juice
- ⅛ tsp Himalayan salt

- 1 ½ cup strawberries, hulled, chopped, and divided
- ½ tbsp fresh mint, thinly sliced
- 1 cup honeydew, diced
- 1 tsp lemon zest
- ⅓ cup almonds, slivered and toasted

Directions:

1. In a food processor, combine the drained cashews, raw honey, vanilla extract, almond extract, lemon juice, and salt. Add half of the strawberries and pulse until everything is combined thoroughly.
2. Pour cashew mixture into serving bowls or glasses and top with remaining strawberries, mint, honeydew, lemon zest, and almonds.
3. Serve immediately.

Nutrition:

- Calories: 11 kcal
- Carbohydrates: 2 g

5. Lettuce & Orange Smoothie

Preparation Time: 5 minutes

Cooking Time: 0 minutes

Servings: 2

Ingredients:

- 1 cup coconut water
- 1 cup lettuce leaves, fresh
- 1 key lime, juiced
- 1 Seville orange, peeled
- 1 tbsp bromide plus powder
- ½ of a medium avocado, pitted

Directions:

1. Take a high-powered blender, switch it on, and then place all the ingredients inside in order.
2. Cover the blender with its lid and then pulse at high speed for 1 minute or more.

Nutrition:

- Calories: 140.5 kcal
- Carbohydrates: 19.7 g
- Fat: 5.5 g
- Fiber: 8.4 g

- Protein: 3.2 g

6. Detox Apple Smoothie

Preparation Time: 5 minutes

Cooking Time: 0 minutes

Servings: 2

Ingredients:

- 2 cups spring water
- 2 cups amaranth greens
- 2 medium fresh apples, cored
- 1 key lime, juiced
- ¼ of avocado

Directions:

1. Take a high-powered blender, switch it on, and then place all the ingredients inside, in order.
2. Cover the blender with its lid and then pulse at high speed for 1 minute or more.

Nutrition:

- Calories: 141 kcal
- Carbohydrates: 27.5 g
- Fat: 2.8 g
- Fiber: 7.5 g
- Protein: 1.4 g

7. Berries & Hemp Seeds Smoothie

Preparation Time: 5 minutes

Cooking Time: 0 minutes

Servings: 2

Ingredients:

- 1 cup spring water
- 2 cups fresh lettuce
- 1 medium banana, peeled
- 1 cup fresh berries, mixed
- 1 Seville orange, peeled
- 1 tbsp hemp seeds
- ¼ of avocado, pitted

Directions:

1. Take a high-powered blender, switch it on, and then place all the ingredients inside in order.
2. Cover the blender with its lid and then pulse at high speed for 1 minute or more.

Nutrition:

- Calories: 216 kcal
- Carbohydrates: 36.2 g
- Fat: 5.5 g
- Fiber: 10.8 g
- Protein: 5.4 g

8. Pear, Berries & Quinoa Smoothie

Preparation Time: 5 minutes

Cooking Time: 0 minute

Servings: 2

Ingredients:

- 2 cups spring water
- ½ avocado, pitted
- 2 fresh pears, chopped
- ½ cup quinoa, cooked
- ¼ cup fresh whole blueberries

Directions:

1. Take a high-powered blender, switch it on, and then place all the ingredients inside in order.
2. Cover the blender with its lid and then pulse at high speed for 1 minute or more.

Nutrition:

- Calories: 325.5 kcal
- Carbohydrates: 57 g
- Fat:7.6 g
- Fiber: 11.4 g
- Protein: 7.3 g

9. Chia Seed Pudding

Preparation Time: 5 hours

Cooking Time: 0 minutes

Servings: 2

Ingredients:

- 3 oz chia seeds
- 1 oz almonds, soaked

- 1 cup low-fat hemp milk
- 2 oz figs
- 1 tsp liquid stevia

Directions:

1. Chop the almonds and put them in 2 mason jars.
2. Then add chia seeds, liquid stevia, and figs.
3. After this, add hemp milk and stir the mixture well.
4. Seal the lids and place the meal in the fridge.
5. Leave the chia pudding in the fridge for at least 5 hours.
6. Enjoy!

Nutrition:

- Calories: 360 kcal
- Fat: 23.8 g
- Carbs: 28.6 g
- Protein: 12.8 g

10.   Scrambled Eggs

Preparation Time: 8 minutes

Cooking Time: 0 minutes

Servings: 4

Ingredients:

- 4 eggs, whisked
- 2 oz watercress
- 4 slices rye bread, gluten-free
- 3 tsp low-fat almond milk
- 1 tsp olive oil
- 1 pinch salt

Directions:

1. Mix up together the whisked eggs and almond milk. Add salt and stir it gently.
2. Place the olive oil in the frying pan and preheat it.
3. After this, add the whisked egg mixture and cook it for 1 minute over medium-high heat.
4. After this, stir the eggs well (scramble them) and cook for 30 seconds more.
5. Scramble the eggs one more time and cook with the closed lid for 2 minutes more over low heat.
6. After cooking the scrambled eggs, transfer them over the rye bread slices and add the watercress.

7. Serve!

Nutrition:

- Calories: 102 kcal
- Fat: 6.7 g
- Carbs: 4 g
- Protein: 6.6 g

11. Muesli-Style Oatmeal

Preparation Time: 5 minutes

Cooking Time: 0 minutes

Servings: 1

Ingredients:

- 1 cup oatmeal
- 1 cup almond milk
- 2 tbsp raisins
- 1 apple, peeled, diced
- Pinch salt
- 2 tsp Splenda

Directions:

1. Soak oatmeal in milk along with salt, Splenda, and raisins in a glass bowl.
2. Cover and refrigerate the bowl for 2 hours.
3. Stir in apples.
4. Serve.

Nutrition:

- Calories: 519 kcal
- Total Fat: 31.4 g
- Saturated Fat: 25.9 g
- Cholesterol: 0 mg
- Sodium: 99 mg
- Carbohydrates: 57.8 g
- Fiber: 8.7 g
- Sugar: 2.3 g
- Protein: 6.5 g

12. Steel Cut Oatmeal

Preparation Time: 15 minutes

Cooking Time: 35 minutes

Servings: 1

Ingredients:

- 1 tbsp almond butter
- 1 cup steel-cut oat
- 3 cups boiling water
- ½ cup almond milk
- ½ cup plus 1 tbsp cashew milk
- 1 tbsp Splenda
- ¼ tsp cinnamon

Directions:

1. Heat almond butter with oats in a saucepan. Stir cook for 2 minutes, then stirs in boiling water. Bring the mixture to a low simmer and cook for 25 minutes.
2. Add half of the almond milk and cashew milk and cook for 10 minutes.
3. Stir in all the remaining ingredients and serve.

Nutrition:

- Calories: 412 kcal
- Total Fat: 24.8 g
- Saturated Fat: 12.4 g
- Cholesterol: 3 mg
- Sodium: 132 mg
- Carbohydrates: 43.8 g
- Dietary Fiber: 13.9 g
- Sugar: 21.5 g
- Protein: 18.9 g

13. Banana Pancakes

Preparation Time: 15 minutes

Cooking Time: 8 minutes

Servings: 2

Ingredients:

- ¼ cup oats, rolled
- ¼ cup arrowroot flour
- ½ tsp organic baking powder
- ¼ tsp organic baking soda
- $\frac{1}{8}$ tsp cinnamon, ground
- ¼ cup almond milk, unsweetened
- 2 organic egg whites
- 2 tsp almond butter
- ½ banana, peeled and mashed well
- $\frac{1}{8}$ tsp organic vanilla extract
- 1 tsp olive oil
- ½ banana, peeled and sliced

Directions:

1. In a large bowl, add the flour, oats, baking soda, baking powder, and cinnamon and mix well.
2. In another bowl, add the almond milk, egg whites, almond butter, mashed banana, and vanilla and beat until well combined.
3. Add the flour mixture and mix until well combined.
4. In a large frying pan, heat the oil over medium-low heat.
5. Add half of the mixture and cook for about 1–2 minutes.
6. Flip to the other side and cook for 1–2 minutes more.
7. Repeat with the remaining mixture.
8. Serve topped with banana slices.

Nutrition:

- Calories: 244 kcal
- Total Fat: 12.7 g
- Saturated Fat: 1.3 g
- Cholesterol: 0 mg
- Sodium: 222 mg
- Carbohydrates: 26.6 g
- Fiber: 4.6 g
- Sugar: 8.3 g
- Protein: 9.8 g

14. Mango Salsa

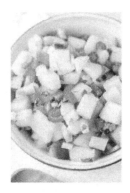

Preparation Time: 15 minutes

Cooking Time: 0 minutes

Servings: 6

Ingredients:

- 1 avocado, peeled, pitted, and cut into cubes
- 2 tbsp fresh lime juice

- 1 mango, peeled, pitted, and cubed
- 1 cup cherry tomatoes, halved
- 1 jalapeño pepper, seeded and chopped
- 1 tbsp fresh cilantro, chopped
- Sea salt, to taste

Directions:

1. Add the avocado and lime juice to a large bowl and mix well.
2. Add the remaining ingredients and stir to combine.
3. Serve immediately.

Nutrition:

- Calories: 108 kcal
- Total Fat: 6.8 g
- Saturated Fat: 1.4 g
- Cholesterol: 0 mg
- Sodium: 43 mg
- Carbohydrates: 12.6 g
- Fiber: 3.6 g
- Sugar: 8.7 g
- Protein: 1.4 g

15. Avocado Gazpacho

Preparation Time: 15 minutes

Cooking Time: 0 minutes

Servings: 6

Ingredients:

- 3 large avocados, peeled, pitted, and chopped
- ⅓ cup fresh cilantro leaves
- 3 cups homemade vegetable broth
- 2 tbsp fresh lemon juice
- 1 tsp cumin, ground
- ¼ tsp cayenne pepper
- Sea salt, to taste

Directions:

1. Add all the ingredients to a high-speed blender and pulse until smooth.
2. Transfer the soup to a large bowl.
3. Cover the bowl and refrigerate to chill for at least 2–3 hours before serving.

Nutrition:

- Calories: 227 kcal
- Total Fat: 20.4 g
- Saturated Fat: 4.4 g
- Cholesterol: 0 mg
- Sodium: 429 mg
- Carbohydrates: 9.4 g
- Fiber: 6.8 g
- Sugar: 1 g
- Protein: 4.5 g

16. Mango Banana Smoothie

Preparation Time: 15 minutes

Cooking Time: 0 minutes

Servings: 1

Ingredients:

- 1 cup spring water
- 2 cups greens
- ½ banana, peeled
- 1 fresh mango, peeled, destoned, sliced

Directions:

1. Take a high-powered blender, switch it on, and then place all the ingredients inside, in order.
2. Cover the blender with its lid and then pulse at high speed for 1 minute.

Nutrition:

- Calories: 95 kcal
- Fiber: 6 g
- Protein: 10 g

17. Toxin Flush Smoothie

Preparation Time: 15 minutes

Cooking Time: 0 minutes

Servings: 1

Ingredients:

- A key lime
- A cucumber
- 1 cup watermelon, cubed, seeded

Directions:

1. Wash and dice the cucumber. Add the watermelon and cucumber to the blender and mix until combined. You shouldn't need to add extra water since both the watermelon and cucumber are mainly water.
2. Slice the lime in half and squeeze the juice into your smoothie. Enjoy.

Nutrition:

- Calories: 111 kcal
- Fiber: 4 g
- Sugar: 1 g

18. Berry Peach Smoothie

Preparation Time: 5 minutes

Cooking Time: 5 minutes

Servings: 2

Ingredients:

- 1 cup coconut water
- 1 tbsp hemp seeds
- 1 tbsp agave
- ½ cup strawberries
- ½ cup blueberries
- ½ cup cherries
- ½ cup peaches

Directions:

1. Place all the ingredients into a blender, then blend until they become smooth and creamy.
2. Serve.

Nutrition:

- Calories: 98 kcal
- Fiber: 6 g
- Sugar: 2 g

19. Veggie Avocado Smoothie

Preparation Time: 5 minutes

Cooking Time: 5 minutes

Servings: 3

Ingredients:

- 1 cup water
- ½ Seville orange, peeled

- 1 avocado
- 1 cucumber, peeled
- 1 cup kale
- 1 cup ice cubes

Directions:

1. Place all the ingredients into a blender, then process until they are smooth and creamy. Serve and enjoy.

Nutrition:

- Calories: 104 kcal
- Fiber: 4 g
- Protein: 9 g

20. Apple Blueberry Smoothie

Preparation Time: 15 minutes

Cooking Time: 0 minutes

Servings: 1

Ingredients:

- ½ apple
- 1 date
- ½ cup blueberries
- ½ cup sparkling callaloo
- 1 tbsp hemp seeds
- 1 tbsp sesame seeds
- 2 cups sparkling soft-jelly coconut water
- ½ tbsp bromide plus powder

Directions:

1. Mix all the ingredients in a high-speed blender. Serve and enjoy!

Nutrition:

- Calories: 98 kcal
- Sugar: 3 g
- Protein: 17 g

21. Alkaline Papaya Smoothie

Preparation Time: 10 minutes

Cooking Time: 0 minutes

Servings: 2

Ingredients:

- ½ large papaya, with seeds
- 4–5 dates
- 2 burro bananas
- ½ lb fresh spring water
- 1 tbsp Bromide Plus Powder
- Juice of ½ a key lime

Directions:

1. To make your alkaline mineral shake, mix all the ingredients in the blender and blend. Add to serving glasses.
2. Serve and enjoy.

Nutrition:

- Calories: 101 kcal
- Fat: 3.6 g
- Protein: 1 g
- Carbohydrates: 17.1 g

22. Heart-Healthy Berry Smoothie

Preparation Time: 15 minutes

Cooking Time: 0 minutes

Servings: 2

Ingredients:

- 1 tbsp Bromide Plus Powder
- ½ lb strawberries
- ½ lb blueberries
- ½ lb blackberries
- ½ lb raspberries
- ½ lb walnuts

Directions:

1. Mix all the ingredients in a high-speed mixer.
2. Add into a serving glass.
3. Serve and enjoy.

Nutrition:

- Calories: 83 kcal
- Total Fat: 5.1 g
- Protein: 2.8 g
- Carbohydrates: 9.1 g

23. Watermelon Smoothie

Preparation Time: 5 minutes

Cooking Time: 0 minutes

Servings: 2

Ingredients:

- 4 cups watermelon, deseeded, cubed
- 4 key limes, juiced
- 4 cucumbers, deseeded, sliced

Directions:

1. Take a high-powered blender, switch it on, and then place all the ingredients inside, in order.
2. Cover the blender with its lid and then pulse at high speed for 1 minute or more.

Nutrition:

- Calories: 123 kcal
- Carbohydrates: 26.1 g
- Fat: 0.8 g
- Fiber: 6.2 g
- Protein: 2.5 g

24. Breakfast Porridge

Preparation Time: 10 minutes

Cooking Time: 50 minutes

Servings: 2

Ingredients:

- ½ cup red or wild rice
- ½ cup steel-cut oats
- ¼ cup pearl barley
- 1 cinnamon stick
- 1–2 tbsp Splenda
- ¼ tsp salt
- ¼ cup fruit, dried (cranberries, cherries, raisins)
- Nuts, chopped, maple syrup and/or milk, for serving (optional)

Directions:

1. Soak rice, barley, farina, and oats in 5 cups of water in a rice cooker.
2. Add cinnamon stick, Splenda, orange peel, salt, and dried fruit.
3. Cover the cooker and cook for 50 minutes on 'manual' functions. Serve with nuts.

Nutrition:

- Calories: 331 kcal
- Total Fat: 2.5 g
- Saturated Fat: 0.5 g
- Cholesterol: 0 mg
- Sodium: 595 mg
- Carbohydrates: 69 g
- Fiber: 12.2 g
- Sugar: 12.5 g
- Protein: 8.7 g

25. Mushroom Omelet With Bell Pepper

Preparation Time: 10 minutes

Cooking Time: 10 minutes

Servings: 2

Ingredients:

- 2 tbsp extra-virgin olive oil
- 1 red bell pepper, sliced
- 1 cup sliced mushrooms
- 6 eggs, beaten
- ½ tsp sea salt
- ⅛ Teaspoon freshly ground black pepper

Directions:

1. Heat the olive oil in a large non-stick skillet over medium-high heat until it shimmers.
2. Add the red bell pepper and mushrooms. Cook for about 4 minutes, occasionally stirring, until soft.
3. In a medium bowl, whisk the eggs, salt, and pepper. Pour the eggs over the vegetables and cook for about 3 minutes without stirring until the eggs begin to set around the edges.
4. Using a rubber spatula, gently pull the eggs away from the edges of the pan. Tilt the pan so the uncooked egg can flow to the edges. Cook for 2–3 minutes until the eggs are set at the edges and the center.
5. Using a spatula, fold the omelet in half. Cut into wedges to serve.

Nutrition:

- Calories: 336
- Fat: 27 g
- Protein: 18 g

- Carbs: 7 g
- Fiber: 1 g
- Sugar: 5 g
- Sodium: 656 mg

26.   Scrambled Eggs With Smoked Salmon

Preparation Time: 5 minutes

Cooking Time: 8 minutes

Servings: 4

Ingredients:

- 2 tbsp extra-virgin olive oil
- 6 oz (170 g) smoked salmon, flaked
- 8 eggs, beaten
- ¼ tsp freshly ground black pepper

Directions:

1. Heat the olive oil in a large non-stick skillet over medium-high heat until it shimmers.
2. Add the salmon and cook for 3 minutes, stirring.
3. In a medium bowl, whisk the eggs and pepper. Add them to the skillet and cook for about 5 minutes, stirring gently, until done.

Nutrition:

- Calories: 236
- Fat: 18 g
- Protein: 19 g
- Carbs: 0 g
- Fiber: 0 g
- Sugar: 0 g
- Sodium: 974 mg

27.   Scotch Eggs With Ground Turkey

Preparation Time: 10 minutes

Cooking Time: 25 minutes

Servings: 2

Ingredients:

- 16 oz (454 g) lean ground turkey
- ½ tsp black pepper

- ½ tsp nutmeg
- ½ tsp cinnamon
- ½ tsp cloves
- ½ tsp dried tarragon
- ½ cup finely chopped fresh parsley
- ½ tbsp dried chives
- 1 clove garlic, finely chopped
- 4 free-range eggs, boiled and peeled

Directions:

1. Preheat the oven to 375°F (190°C).
2. Cover a baking sheet with parchment paper.
3. Combine the turkey with the cinnamon, nutmeg, pepper, cloves, tarragon, chives, parsley, and garlic in a mixing bowl and mix with your hands until thoroughly mixed.
4. Divide the mixture into 4 circular shapes with the palms of your hands.
5. Flatten each one into a pancake shape using the backs of your hands or a rolling pin.
6. Wrap the meat pancake around 1 egg, until it's covered. (You can moisten the meat with water first to help prevent it from sticking to your hands).
7. Bake in the oven for 25 minutes or until brown and crisp.
8. Serve and enjoy!

Nutrition:

- Calories: 502
- Fat: 30 g
- Protein: 55 g
- Carbs: 3 g
- Fiber: 1 g
- Sugar: 1 g
- Sodium: 290 mg

28.   Green Berry Smoothie

Preparation Time: 10 minutes

Cooking Time: 0 minutes

Servings: 2

Ingredients:

- 1 handful Kale leaves
- 1 cup blueberries
- 2 tbsp lime juice
- 1 tbsp sea moss

- 1 tbsp hemp seeds
- 1 cup coconut milk

Directions:

1. Pour all ingredients into a blender. Blend for 30 seconds at a time until the mixture is smooth.
2. You may dilute with water to derive the desired thickness.

Nutrition:

- Calories: 118 kcal
- Protein: 25 g
- Fiber: 17 g
- Sugar: 8 g

29. Apple Berry Smoothie

Preparation Time: 10 minutes

Cooking Time: 0 minutes

Servings: 2

Ingredients:

- 1 handful kale leaves
- 1 cup blueberries
- 2 tbsp lime juice
- 1 tbsp sea moss
- 1 tbsp hemp seeds
- 1 cup coconut milk

Directions:

1. Pour all ingredients into a blender. Blend for 30 seconds at a time until the mixture is smooth.
2. You may dilute with water to derive the desired thickness.

Nutrition:

- Calories: 209 kcal
- Protein: 30 g
- Fiber: 24 g
- Sugar: 9 g

30. Watermelon Detox Smoothie

Preparation Time: 10 minutes

Cooking Time: 0 minutes

Servings: 2

Ingredients:

- ½ watermelon, chopped into bits
- ¼ cup grape juice with seeds
- 1 peach, chopped into bits

Directions:

1. Pour all ingredients into a blender. Blend for 30 seconds at a time until the mixture is smooth.
2. You may dilute with water to derive the desired thickness.

Nutrition:

- Calories: 128 kcal
- Protein: 22 g
- Fiber: 14 g
- Sugar: 4 g

Chapter 3. Lunch Recipes

31. Buckwheat Salad

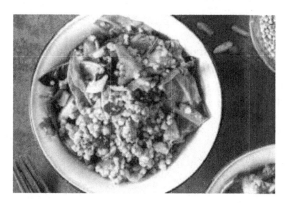

Preparation Time: 10 minutes

Cooking Time: 15 minutes

Servings: 2

Ingredients:

- 1 cup raw buckwheat, rinsed
- 2 cups water
- 2 handfuls fresh baby spinach leaves, rinsed
- Handful fresh basil leaves, rinsed
- 2 scallions, white parts only, rinsed and chopped
- Zest 1 lemon
- Juice ½ lemon
- ½ red onion, finely chopped
- Himalayan pink salt to taste
- Black pepper, freshly ground to taste
- ¼ cup extra-virgin olive oil
- 1 red chili, rinsed and thinly sliced
- 2 tbsp mixed sprouts, rinsed
- 1 ripe avocado, peeled, pitted, and sliced
- 1½ oz feta cheese (optional)

Directions:

1. Mix the buckwheat and water, then bring it to a boil over high heat. Reduce the heat to simmer and cook for 15 minutes or until soft. Remove from the heat and let cool.
2. Meanwhile, in a food processor, combine the baby spinach, basil, scallions, lemon zest, and lemon juice, and process for 30 seconds. Stir the herb mixture into the cooled buckwheat.
3. Add the red onion and season with salt and pepper.

4. Arrange the buckwheat on a platter. Drizzle with the olive oil and scatter on the chopped chili and sprouts. Top with the sliced avocado, crumble the feta over the top (if using), and serve.

Nutrition:

- Calories: 685 kcal
- Total Fat: 54 g
- Total Carbohydrates: 43 g
- Fiber: 16 g
- Sugar: 5 g

32. Mixed Sprouts Salad

Preparation Time: 10 minutes

Cooking Time: 0 minutes

Servings: 2

Ingredients:

- 1–2 tbsp coconut oil
- Juice of 1 lemon
- Handful fresh chives, rinsed and chopped
- Handful fresh dill, rinsed and chopped
- Handful fresh parsley, rinsed and chopped
- ½ tsp Himalayan pink salt
- ½ tsp black pepper, freshly ground
- 1 scallion, rinsed and chopped
- 1 cucumber, rinsed and chopped
- ½ cup mixed sprouts of choice (alfalfa, radish, broccoli, mung bean, cress, etc.), rinsed

Directions:

1. In a blender, combine the coconut oil, lemon juice, chives, dill, parsley, salt, and pepper, and blend until mainly smooth. Transfer to a medium bowl. Stir in the scallion, cucumber, and sprouts to coat, and serve.

Nutrition:

- Calories: 168 kcal
- Total Fat:14 g
- Total Carbohydrates: 12 g
- Fiber: 1 g
- Sugar: 4 g

33. Thai Quinoa Salad

Preparation Time: 15 minutes

Cooking Time: 0 minutes

Servings: 2

Ingredients:

For the dressing:

- ⅓ cup water, filtered
- ¼ cup tahini
- 1 date, pitted
- 1 tbsp sesame seeds
- 1 tbsp apple cider vinegar
- 2 tsp tamari
- 1 tsp lemon juice, freshly squeezed
- 1 tsp sesame oil, toasted
- 1 tsp garlic, chopped
- ½ tsp Himalayan pink salt

For the salad:

- 1 cup quinoa, rinsed and steamed
- 1 cup arugula, rinsed and chopped
- 1 tomato, rinsed and sliced
- ¼ red onion, rinsed and diced

Directions:

To make the dressing:

1. Blend the water, tahini, date, sesame seeds, vinegar, tamari, lemon juice, sesame oil, garlic, and salt at high speed until smooth.

To make the salad:

1. Combine together the quinoa, arugula, tomato, and red onion. Drizzle the dressing, toss it well to coat, and serve.

Nutrition:

- Calories: 558 kcal
- Total Fat: 25 g
- Total Carbohydrates: 69 g
- Fiber: 10 g
- Sugar: 4 g
- Protein: 19 g

34. Sweet Potato Salad

Preparation Time: 15 minutes

Cooking Time: 5 minutes

Servings: 2

Ingredients:

For the dressing:

- ½ cup sesame oil
- 2 tbsp coconut oil
- 2 tbsp light soy sauce
- 1 tbsp coconut sugar or raw honey
- 1 garlic clove, crushed

For the salad:

- 5 ½ oz fresh baby spinach leaves, rinsed
- 1 red onion, rinsed and finely chopped
- 1 tomato, rinsed, seeded, and chopped
- 1 tbsp coconut oil
- 1 large sweet potato, scrubbed, peeled, and diced

Directions:

To make the dressing:

1. In a small bowl, whisk the sesame oil, coconut oil, soy sauce, coconut sugar, and garlic until blended. Set aside.

To make the salad:

1. In a large salad bowl, gently toss together the baby spinach, red onion, and tomato. Set aside.
2. In a small skillet over medium heat, heat the coconut oil. Add the sweet potato and cook for 3–5 minutes, stirring, until golden brown.
3. Add the sweet potato to the salad using a slotted spoon and gently stir to combine. Pour the dressing over the salad, gently toss again to coat, and serve.

Nutrition:

- Calories: 550 kcal
- Total Fat: 52 g
- Total Carbohydrates: 20 g
- Fiber: 3 g
- Sugar: 9 g

35. Waldorf Salad

Preparation Time: 15 minutes plus overnight to soak

Cooking Time: 0 minutes

Servings: 2

Ingredients:

For the dressing:

- 1 ripe avocado, peeled and pitted
- 1 tsp Dijon mustard
- ½ tsp Himalayan pink salt
- Freshly ground black pepper
- Juice of ½ lemon

For the salad:

- 2 cups chickpeas, canned, rinsed and drained, or cooked, drained, and cooled
- 1 cup sunflower seeds, soaked in filtered water overnight, drained
- 2 apples, rinsed, cored, and chopped
- ½ red onion, rinsed and diced
- 1 celery stalk, rinsed and diced
- 1–2 tsp fresh dill, chopped and rinsed

Directions:

To make the dressing:

1. Using a fork, mash together the avocado, mustard, salt, pepper, and lemon juice in a small bowl.
2. Set aside.

To make the salad:

1. In a large bowl, stir the chickpeas, sunflower seeds, and dressing until well combined. Stir in the apples, red onion, and celery.
2. Top with the fresh dill and serve.

Nutrition:

- Calories: 700 kcal
- Total Fat:40 g
- Total Carbohydrates: 80 g
- Fiber: 28 g
- Protein: 28 g

36. Vegetable Stuffed Quinoa With Steamed Zucchini

Preparation Time: 10 minutes

Cooking Time: 15 minutes

Servings: 2–4

Ingredients:

- 1 cup quinoa
- 1 ½ cup water
- 2 tbsp coconut milk
- ¾ cup mushrooms, chopped
- 1-inch section red bell pepper, chopped
- ¼ onion, chopped
- 1 plum tomato, chopped
- ½ tsp sea salt
- Spices: a dash of basil, oregano, thyme, red pepper flakes
- ⅓ zucchini, sliced

Directions:

1. Dip the quinoa for at least 5 minutes, strain, and rinse to remove wax.
2. Add all the ingredients (except for the zucchini) to a saucepan and bring to a boil.
3. Lower the heat, then simmer until the water is absorbed.
4. Steam the zucchini slices in a steamer for 5–10 minutes.
5. Plate and serve.

Nutrition:

- Calories: 104 kcal
- Protein: 5.8 g
- Fiber: 2.1 g

37. Garlic & Shrimp Pasta

Preparation Time: 4 minutes

Cooking Time: 16 minutes

Servings: 4

Ingredients:

- 6 oz whole-wheat spaghetti
- 12 oz raw shrimp, peeled and deveined, cut into 1-inch pieces
- 1 bunch asparagus, trimmed
- 1 large bell pepper, thinly sliced
- 1 cup fresh peas
- 3 garlic cloves, chopped
- 1 and ¼ tsp kosher salt
- ½ and ½ cup non-fat plain yogurt
- 3 tbsp lemon juice
- 1 tbsp extra-virgin olive oil
- ½ tsp fresh ground black pepper

- ¼ cup pine nuts, toasted

Directions:

1. Take a large-sized pot and bring water to a boil.
2. Add your spaghetti and cook them for about minutes less than the directed package instruction.
3. Add shrimp, bell pepper, asparagus, and cook for about 2–4 minutes until the shrimp are tender.
4. Drain the pasta and the contents well.
5. Take a large bowl and mash the garlic until it forms a paste.
6. Whisk in yogurt, parsley, oil, pepper, and lemon juice into the garlic paste.
7. Add pasta, mix, and toss well.
8. Serve by sprinkling some pine nuts!

Nutrition:

- Calories: 406 kcal
- Fat: 22 g
- Protein: 26 g

38.   Paprika Butter Shrimps

Preparation Time: 6 minutes

Cooking Time: 31 minutes

Servings: 2

Ingredients:

- ¼ tbsp paprika, smoked
- ⅛ cup sour cream
- ½ lb tiger shrimps
- ⅛ cup butter
- Salt and black pepper, to taste

Directions:

1. Prep the oven to 390°F and grease a baking dish.
2. Mix all the ingredients in a large bowl and transfer them to the baking dish.
3. Situate in the oven and bake for about 15 minutes.
4. Place paprika shrimp in a dish and set aside to cool for meal prepping. Divide it into 2 containers and cover the lid. Refrigerate for 1–2 days and reheat in the microwave before serving.

Nutrition:

- Calories: 330 kcal
- Protein: 32.6 g
- Fat: 21.5 g

39.   Tuna With Vegetable Mix

Preparation Time: 8 minutes

Cooking Time: 16 minutes

Servings: 4

Ingredients:

- ¼ cup extra-virgin olive oil, divided
- 1 tbsp rice vinegar
- 1 tsp kosher salt, divided
- ¾ tsp Dijon mustard
- ¾ tsp honey
- 4 oz baby gold beets, thinly sliced
- 4 oz fennel bulb, trimmed and thinly sliced
- 4 oz baby turnips, thinly sliced
- 6 oz Granny Smith apple, very thinly sliced
- 2 tsp sesame seeds, toasted
- 6 oz tuna steaks
- ½ tsp black pepper
- 1 tbsp fennel fronds, torn

Directions:

1. Scourge 2 tbsp of oil, ½ tsp of salt, honey, vinegar, and mustard.
2. Give the mixture a nice mix.
3. Add fennel, beets, apple, and turnips; mix and toss until everything is evenly coated.
4. Sprinkle with sesame seeds and toss well.
5. Using a cast-iron skillet, heat 2 tbsp of oil over high heat.
6. Carefully season the tuna with ½ tsp of salt and pepper.
7. Situate the tuna in the skillet and cook for 4 minutes, giving 1½ minutes per side.
8. Remove the tuna and slice it up.
9. Place in containers with the vegetable mix.
10. Serve with the fennel mix, and enjoy!

Nutrition:

- Calories: 443 kcal
- Fat: 17.1 g
- Protein: 16.5 g

40.   Chicken & Butter Sauce

Preparation Time: 5 minutes

Cooking Time: 30 minutes

Servings: 5

Ingredients:

- 1-lb chicken fillet
- ⅓ cup butter, softened
- 1 tbsp rosemary
- ½ tsp thyme
- 1 tsp salt
- ½ lemon

Directions:

1. Churn together thyme, salt, and rosemary.
2. Chop the chicken fillet roughly and mix it up with churned butter mixture.
3. Place the prepared chicken in the baking dish.
4. Squeeze the lemon over the chicken.
5. Chop the squeezed lemon and add it to the baking dish.
6. Cover the chicken with foil and bake it for 20 minutes at 365°F.
7. Then discard the foil and bake the chicken for 10 minutes more.

Nutrition:

- Calories: 285 kcal
- Fat: 19.1 g
- Fiber: 0.5 g
- Carbs: 1 g
- Protein: 26.5 g

41.Pork & Chestnuts Mix

Preparation Time: 30 minutes

Cooking Time: 0 minutes

Servings: 6

Ingredients:

- 1½ cup brown rice, already cooked
- 2 cups pork roast, already cooked and shredded
- 3 oz water chestnuts, drained and sliced
- ½ cup sour cream

- A pinch salt and white pepper

Directions:

1. Mix the rice with the roast and other ingredients in a bowl, toss and keep in the fridge for 2 hours before serving.

Nutrition:

- Calories: 294 kcal
- Fat: 17 g
- Fiber: 8 g
- Carbs: 16 g
- Protein: 23.5 g

42.   Greek Baked Cod

Preparation Time: 9 minutes

Cooking Time: 13 minutes

Servings: 4

Ingredients:

- 1 ½ lb Cod fillet pieces (4–6 pieces)
- 5 garlic cloves, peeled and minced
- ¼ cup fresh parsley leaves, chopped
- Lemon Juice Mixture:
- 5 tbsp fresh lemon juice
- 5 tbsp extra virgin olive oil
- 2 tbsp vegan butter, melted

For coating:

- ⅓ cup all-purpose flour
- 1 tsp coriander, ground
- ¾ tsp sweet Spanish paprika
- ¾ tsp cumin, ground
- ¾ tsp salt
- ½ tsp black pepper

Directions:

1. Preheat the oven to 400°F.
2. Scourge lemon juice, olive oil, and melted butter, set aside.
3. Mix all-purpose flour, spices, salt, and pepper in another shallow bowl, and set next to the lemon bowl to create a station.
4. Pat the fish fillet dry, then dip the fish in the lemon juice mixture, then dip it in the flour mixture, and brush off extra flour.

5. In a cast-iron skillet over medium-high heat, add 2 tbsp olive oil.
6. Once heated, add in the fish and sear on each side for color, but do not thoroughly cook; remove from heat.
7. With the remaining lemon juice mixture, add the minced garlic and mix.
8. Drizzle all over the fish fillets.
9. Bake for 10 minutes, until it begins to flake easily with a fork.
10. Allow the dish to cool completely.
11. Distribute among the containers, and store for 2–3 days.
12. To Serve: Reheat in the microwave for 1–2 minutes or until heated through. Sprinkle chopped parsley. Enjoy!

Nutrition:

- Calories: 321 kcal
- Fat: 18 g
- Protein: 23 g

43. Pistachio Sole Fish

Preparation Time: 4 minutes

Cooking Time: 11 minutes

Servings: 4

Ingredients:

- 4 (5 oz) sole fillets, boneless
- Salt and pepper, as needed
- ½ cup pistachios, finely chopped
- Zest of 1 lemon
- Juice of 1 lemon
- 1 tsp extra virgin olive oil

Directions:

1. Preheat your oven to 350°F.
2. Prep a baking sheet using parchment paper, then keep aside.
3. Pat fish dry with kitchen towels and lightly season with salt and pepper.
4. Take a small bowl and stir in pistachios and lemon zest.
5. Place sole on the prepped sheet and press 2 tbsp of the pistachio mixture on top of each fillet.
6. Rub fish with lemon juice and olive oil.
7. Bake for 10 minutes until the top is golden and fish flakes with a fork.

8. Serve and enjoy!

Meal Prep/Storage Options: Store in airtight containers in your fridge for 1–2 days.

Nutrition:

- Calories: 166 kcal
- Fat: 6 g
- Protein: 26 g

44. Baked Tilapia

Preparation Time: 9 minutes

Cooking Time: 16 minutes

Servings: 4

Ingredients:

- 1 lb tilapia fillets (about 8 fillets)
- 1 tsp olive oil
- 1 tbsp vegan butter
- 2 shallots, finely chopped
- 3 garlic cloves, minced
- 1 ½ tsp cumin, ground
- 1 ½ tsp paprika
- ¼ cup capers
- ¼ cup fresh dill, finely chopped
- Juice from 1 lemon
- Salt and pepper to taste

Directions:

1. Preheat the oven to 375°F.
2. Prep a rimmed baking sheet using parchment paper or foil.
3. Lightly mist with cooking spray, and arrange the fish fillets evenly on the baking sheet.
4. Mix the cumin, paprika, salt, and pepper.
5. Rub the fish fillets with the spice mixture.
6. Scourge the melted butter, lemon juice, shallots, olive oil, and garlic, and brush evenly over fish fillets.
7. Top with the capers.
8. Bake for 13 minutes.
9. Pull out from the oven and allow the dish to cool completely.
10. Distribute among the containers, and store for 2–3 days.

11. To serve: Reheat in the microwave for 1–2 minutes or until heated through. Top with fresh dill. Serve!

Nutrition:

- Calories: 410 kcal
- Fat: 5 g
- Protein: 21 g

45.   A Great Mediterranean Snapper

Preparation Time: 11 minutes

Cooking Time: 19 minutes

Servings: 2

Ingredients:

- 2 tbsp extra virgin olive oil
- 1 medium onion, chopped
- 2 garlic cloves, minced
- 1 tsp oregano
- 1 can (14 oz) tomatoes, diced with juice
- ½ cup black olives, sliced
- 4 red snapper fillets (each 4 oz
- Salt and pepper, as needed

Garnish:

- ¼ cup feta cheese, crumbled
- ¼ cup parsley, minced

Directions:

1. Preheat your oven to a temperature of 425°F.
2. Take a 13x9 inch baking dish and grease it up with non-stick cooking spray.
3. Take a large-sized skillet and place it over medium heat.
4. Add oil and heat it up.
5. Add onion, oregano, and garlic.
6. Sauté for 2 minutes.
7. Add diced tomatoes with juice alongside black olives.
8. Bring the mix to a boil.
9. Remove the heat.
10. Place the fish on the prepped baking dish.
11. Season both sides with salt and pepper.
12. Spoon the tomato mix over the fish.
13. Bake for 10 minutes.

14. Remove the oven and sprinkle a bit of parsley and feta.
15. Enjoy!

Nutrition:

- Calories: 269 kcal
- Fat: 13 g
- Protein: 27 g

46.   Stuffed Bell Peppers

Preparation Time: 10 minutes

Cooking Time: 15 minutes

Servings: 1–2

Ingredients:

- 1 cup quinoa
- 1½ cup water
- 2 green bell peppers
- 1 lb oyster or another mushroom
- 1 tbsp grapeseed or avocado oil
- ½ red bell pepper chopped fine
- ½ tsp basil
- ½ tsp dill
- ½ tsp sea salt
- ⅛ tsp cayenne pepper

Directions:

1. Soak quinoa for 5–10 minutes and rinse.
2. Combine quinoa and water in a saucepan. Let it boil, then adjust the heat to low and cook for 15–20 minutes. Set aside.
3. Remove the stem, cut off the tops, and hollow out the green bell peppers.
4. Steam in a steamer until softened.
5. Sauté mushrooms in oil over medium heat. It is important not to cook on high heat to maintain the integrity of the oil and food.
6. Remove mushrooms from the pan at let cool.
7. Combine cooked quinoa, mushrooms, and spices and mix.
8. Stuff green bell peppers with e quinoa.
9. Mix and serve.

Nutrition:

- Calories: 98 kcal
- Protein: 7.9 g
- Fiber: 4.8 g

47.   Seasoned Wild Rice

Preparation Time: 5 minutes

Cooking Time: 25 minutes

Servings: 1–2

Ingredients:

- 1 cup wild rice (soak wild rice overnight)
- 2–3 cups water (3 cup water if you didn't soak the rice overnight)
- 1 tbsp coconut oil
- 2 tsp oregano
- ½ tsp sea salt
- ⅛ tsp cayenne pepper
- 2–3 scallions, chopped
- 1 plum tomato, chopped

Directions:

1. Soaking the rice in water overnight reduces the cooking time for the rice.
2. Transfer all the ingredients to a saucepan over high heat and let them come to a boil. Cover the saucepan, reduce to a simmer, and allow the water to absorb into the rice. If you soaked the rice overnight, cook the rice for 25 minutes. If you did not soak the rice overnight, cook for 50–60 minutes.

Nutrition:

- Calories: 150 kcal
- Protein: 25 g
- Fiber: 8 g

48.   Roasted Large Cap Portobello Mushrooms & Yellow Squash

Preparation Time: 10 minutes

Cooking Time: 30 minutes

Servings: 1–2

Ingredients:

- 3 large Portobello mushrooms
- 9 ½ inch slices yellow squash
- Avocado oil (brush on front and back of mushrooms)
- ½ lime

- Spices (coriander, cayenne pepper, oregano, sea salt)

Directions:

1. Pull off the Portobello mushroom stems and scoop out the fins with a spoon. Brush on avocado oil on the front and back of the mushrooms. Squeeze a little lime over the tops of the mushrooms.
2. Sprinkle the spices on the mushrooms and yellow squash but keep the mushrooms and squash separate. Heat oven to 400°F. Place mushrooms on the roasting pan, scooped outside facing up—Cook for 10 minutes.
3. Carefully remove the pan and mushrooms, and add 3 seasoned yellow squash slices to each mushroom top. Put the roasting pan back into the oven. Cook the mushrooms and squash for another 10 minutes. Remove from oven and serve hot.

Nutrition:

- Calories: 108 kcal
- Protein: 5.9 g
- Fiber: 1.7 g

49.   Tuna Bowl With Kale

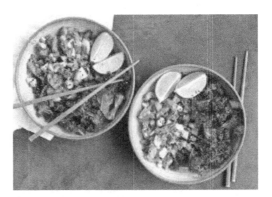

Preparation Time: 4 minutes

Cooking Time: 18 minutes

Servings: 6

Ingredients:

- 3 tbsp extra virgin olive oil
- 1 ½ tsp garlic, minced
- ¼ cup capers
- 2 tsp sugar

- 15 oz can great northern beans, drained and rinsed
- 1-lb kale, chopped with the center ribs removed
- ½ tsp black pepper, ground
- 1 cup onion, chopped
- 2 ½ oz olives, drained and sliced
- ¼ tsp sea salt
- ¼ tsp red pepper, crushed
- 6 oz tuna in olive oil, do not drain

Directions:

1. Place a large pot, like a stockpot, on your stove and turn the burner to high heat.
2. Fill the pot about ¾ of the way full with water and let it come to a boil.
3. Cook the kale for 2 minutes.
4. Drain the kale and set it aside.
5. Set the heat to medium and place the empty pot back on the burner.
6. Add the oil and onion. Sauté for 3–4 minutes.
7. Combine the garlic into the oil mixture and sauté for another minute.
8. Add the capers, olives, and red pepper.
9. Cook the ingredients for another minute while stirring.
10. Pour in the sugar and stir while you toss in the kale. Mix all the ingredients thoroughly and ensure the kale is thoroughly coated.
11. Cover the pot and set the timer for 8 minutes.
12. Put off the heat and stir in the tuna, pepper, beans, salt, and any other herbs that will make this one of the best Mediterranean dishes you've ever made.

Nutrition:

- Calories: 265 kcal
- Fat: 12 g
- Protein: 16 g

50. Chicken & Olives Salsa

Preparation Time: 10 minutes

Cooking Time: 25 minutes

Servings: 4

Ingredients:

- 2 tbsp avocado oil
- 4 chicken breast halves, skinless and boneless

- Salt and black pepper, to the taste
- 1 tbsp sweet paprika
- 1 red onion, chopped
- 1 tbsp balsamic vinegar
- 2 tbsp parsley, chopped
- 1 avocado, peeled, pitted, and cubed
- 2 tbsp black olives, pitted and chopped

Directions:

1. Heat and set your grill over medium-high heat, add the chicken brushed with half of the oil and seasoned with salt, and pepper, cook for 7 minutes on each side, and divide between plates.
2. Meanwhile, mix the onion with the remaining ingredients and the remaining oil in a bowl, toss, add on top of the chicken and serve.

Nutrition:

- Calories: 289 kcal
- Fat: 12.4 g
- Fiber: 9.1 g
- Carbs: 23.8 g
- Protein: 14.3 g

51. Balsamic Chicken

Preparation Time: 10 minutes

Cooking Time: 30 minutes

Servings: 4

Ingredients:

- 3 chicken breasts
- ¼ cup olive oil
- ¼ cup balsamic vinegar
- 1 clove garlic

Directions:

1. In a bowl, add all ingredients.
2. Add chicken and the marinade for 3–4 hours.
3. Grill and serve with vegetables.

Nutrition:

- Calories: 200 kcal
- Fat: 8 g
- Fiber: 4 g
- Carbs: 8 g
- Protein: 3 g

52. Lemon Chicken Mix

Preparation Time: 10 minutes

Cooking Time: 10 minutes

Servings: 2

Ingredients:

- 8 oz chicken breast, skinless, boneless
- 1 tsp Cajun seasoning
- 1 tsp balsamic vinegar
- 1 tsp olive oil
- 1 tsp lemon juice

Directions:

1. Cut the chicken breast into halves and sprinkle with Cajun seasoning.
2. Then sprinkle the poultry with olive oil and lemon juice.
3. Then sprinkle the chicken breast with balsamic vinegar.
4. Preheat the grill to 385°F.
5. Grill the chicken breast halves for 5 minutes from each side.
6. Slice Cajun chicken and place it on the serving plate.

Nutrition:

- Calories: 150 kcal
- Fat: 5.2 g
- Fiber: 0 g
- Carbs: 0.1 g
- Protein: 24.1 g

53. Chicken Shawarma

Preparation Time: 15 minutes

Cooking Time: 30 minutes

Servings: 8

Ingredients:

- 2 lb chicken breast, sliced into strips
- 1 tsp paprika
- 1 tsp cumin, ground
- ¼ tsp garlic, granulated
- ½ tsp turmeric

- ¼ tsp allspice, ground

Directions:

1. Season the chicken with spices and a little salt and pepper.
2. Pour 1 cup of chicken broth into the pot.
3. Seal the pot.
4. Choose a poultry setting.
5. Cook for 15 minutes.
6. Release the pressure naturally.

Nutrition:

- Calories: 132 kcal
- Total Fat: 3 g
- Saturated Fat: 0 g
- Cholesterol: 73 mg
- Sodium: 58 mg
- Total Carbohydrates: 0.5 g
- Dietary Fiber: 0.2 g
- Total Sugar: 0.1 g
- Protein: 24.2 g
- Potassium: 435 mg

54. Lemon Chicken

Preparation Time: 10 minutes

Cooking Time: 20 minutes

Servings: 4

Ingredients:

- 1-lb chicken breast, skinless, boneless
- 3 tbsp lemon juice
- 1 tbsp olive oil
- 1 tsp black pepper, ground

Directions:

1. Cut the chicken breast into 4 pieces.
2. Sprinkle every chicken piece with olive oil, lemon juice, and ground black pepper.
3. Then place them in the skillet.
4. Roast the chicken for 20 minutes over medium heat.
5. Flip the chicken pieces every 5 minutes.

Nutrition:

- Calories: 163 kcal
- Fat: 6.5 g
- Fiber: 0.2 g

- Carbs: 0.6 g
- Protein: 24.2 g

55.   Greek Chicken Bites

Preparation Time: 10 minutes

Cooking Time: 20 minutes

Servings: 6

Ingredients:

- 1-lb chicken fillet
- 1 tbsp Greek seasoning
- 1 tsp sesame oil
- ½ tsp salt
- 1 tsp balsamic vinegar

Directions:

1. Cut the chicken fingers on small tenders (fingers) and sprinkle them with Greek seasoning, salt, and balsamic vinegar. Mix up well with the help of the fingertips.
2. Then sprinkle chicken with sesame oil and shake gently.
3. Line the baking tray with parchment.
4. Place the marinated chicken fingers in the tray in one layer.
5. Bake the chicken fingers for 20 minutes at 355°F. Flip them to another side after 10 minutes of cooking.

Nutrition:

- Calories: 154 kcal
- Fat: 6.4 g
- Fiber: 0 g
- Carbs: 0.8 g
- Protein: 22 g

56.   Turkey Verde With Brown Rice

Preparation Time: 15 minutes

Cooking Time: 30 minutes

Servings: 5

Ingredients:

- ⅔ cup chicken broth

- 1¼ cup brown rice
- 1½ lb turkey tenderloins
- 1 onion, sliced
- ½ cup salsa verde

Directions:

1. Add the chicken broth and rice to the Instant Pot.
2. Top with the turkey, onion, and salsa. Cover the pot.
3. Set it to manual and cook at high pressure for 18 minutes.
4. Release the pressure naturally.
5. Wait for 8 minutes before opening the pot.

Nutrition:

- Calories: 336 kcal
- Total Fat: 3.3 g
- Saturated Fat: 0.3 g
- Cholesterol: 54 mg
- Sodium: 321 mg
- Total Carbohydrates: 39.4 g
- Dietary Fiber: 2.2 g
- Total Sugar: 1.4 g
- Protein: 38.5 g
- Potassium: 187 mg

57. Chicken Tacos

Preparation Time: 10 minutes

Cooking Time: 20 minutes

Servings: 4

Ingredients:

- 2 bread tortillas
- 1 tsp butter
- 2 tsp olive oil
- 1 tsp Taco seasoning
- 6 oz chicken breast, skinless, boneless, sliced
- ⅓ cup Cheddar cheese, shredded
- 1 bell pepper, cut on the wedges

Directions:

1. Pour 1 tsp of olive oil into the skillet and add chicken.
2. Sprinkle the meat with Taco seasoning and mix up well.

3. Roast the chicken for 10 minutes over medium heat.
4. Stir it from time to time.
5. Then transfer the cooked chicken to the plate.
6. Add remaining olive oil to the skillet.
7. Then add bell pepper and roast it for 5 minutes.
8. Stir it all the time.
9. Mix up together bell pepper with chicken.
10. Toss butter in the skillet and melt it.
11. Put 1 tortilla in the skillet.
12. Put Cheddar cheese on the tortilla and flatten it.
13. Then add a chicken-pepper mixture and cover it with the second tortilla.
14. Roast the quesadilla for 2 minutes from each side.
15. Cut the cooked meal into halves and transfer it to the serving plates.

Nutrition:

- Calories: 194 kcal
- Fat: 8.3 g
- Fiber: 0.6 g
- Carbs: 16.4 g
- Protein: 13.2 g

58. Spelt Spaghetti

Preparation Time: 10 minutes

Cooking Time: 20 minutes

Servings: 2–3

Ingredients:

- 1–8 oz box Spelt Spaghetti (Nature's Legacy makes a product that is only made from spelled and water.)

Directions:

1. Boil 2 quarts of water in a pot. Slowly add in the spelled spaghetti.
2. Cook for 10 minutes, stirring occasionally. Don't overcook.
3. Drain and plate.

Nutrition:

- Calories: 87 kcal
- Protein: 6.8 g
- Fiber: 1.5 g

59. Butternut Squash Plum Tomato

Spaghetti Sauce

Preparation Time: 5 minutes

Cooking Time: 20 minutes

Servings: 4

Ingredients:

- ½ butternut squash
- ¼ plum tomato, chopped
- 1 cup water
- Spices: a dash cayenne pepper, onion, basil, bay leaf, oregano, thyme, savory, coriander, and salt

Directions:

1. Add butternut squash cubes to a pot, cover with water and boil until squash becomes tender. Remove squash from water.
2. Add squash, tomato, and spices to a blender and blend; slowly add water until you reach desired consistency.
3. Add to a container, let cool, and refrigerate.

Nutrition:

- Calories: 105 kcal
- Protein: 21 g
- Fiber: 12 g

60. Simply Chayote Squash

Preparation Time: 10 minutes

Cooking Time: 20 minutes

Servings: 1

Ingredients:

- 1 chayote squash
- ¼ tsp coconut oil
- Dash cayenne pepper
- Dash sea salt

Directions:

1. Wash and cut chayote squash in half. The seed can be eaten, and it has a nice texture.
2. Add chayote, oil, and enough water to cover the chayote in a saucepan.

3. Boil for 20 minutes until the fork can penetrate the squash, but the squash should still maintain some firmness.
4. Remove from water. Season it well with cayenne pepper and salt.
5. Serve as a light snack or part of a dish.

Nutrition:

- Calories: 117 kcal
- Fiber: 9.7 g
- Protein: 14 g

61. Vegetable Medley Sauté

Preparation Time: 10 minutes

Cooking Time: 15 minutes

Servings: 4

Ingredients:

- 1 cup mushrooms, sliced
- 1 zucchini, sliced
- 1 yellow squash, sliced
- 1 red pepper, chopped
- 1 green pepper, chopped
- 2 plum tomatoes, chopped
- ½ red onion, finely chopped
- ½ cup chayote, finely chopped
- 3 tbsp grapeseed oil or avocado oil
- ⅛ tsp cayenne pepper
- ⅛ tsp sea salt

Directions:

1. Cook the oil in a saucepan over medium heat. Let the oil get hot.
2. Add in mushrooms and onions and sauté for 4 minutes.
3. Add the rest of the vegetables and spices, and sauté for 8–10 minutes.

Nutrition:

- Calories: 115 kcal
- Fiber: 4.9 g
- Protein: 21 g

62. Chickpea Butternut Squash

Preparation Time: 10 minutes

Cooking Time: 15 minutes

Servings: 2

Ingredients:

- 15 oz chickpeas, cooked
- 1 ½ section of a butternut squash
- ¼ plum tomato
- ¼ cup coconut milk
- 1 cup water (add more water to make thinner soup)
- Pinch dill
- Pinch allspice
- Pinch cayenne pepper
- ⅛ tsp sea salt

Directions:

1. Add all the ingredients to a blender and blend to your desired consistency.
2. Add the blended ingredients to a saucepan over a medium/high flame until it starts to boil or air bubbles rise.
3. Adjust it to low heat and cook for 30 minutes.

Nutrition:

- Calories: 110 kcal
- Fiber: 9.7 g
- Protein: 11 g

Chapter 4. Dinner Recipes

63. Chicken Bone Broth

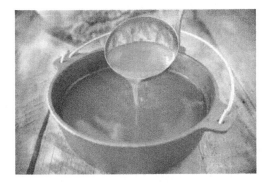

Preparation Time: 10 minutes

Cooking Time: 90 minutes

Servings: 8

Ingredients:

- Bones from a 3 - 4 pounds chicken
- 4 cups water
- 2 large carrots, cut into chunks
- 2 large stalks celery
- 1 large onion
- 4 Fresh rosemary sprigs
- 3 fresh thyme sprigs
- 2 tbsp apple cider vinegar
- 1 tsp kosher salt

Directions:

1. Put all the ingredients and allow it to sit for 30 minutes.
2. Pressure cook and adjust the time to 90 minutes.
3. Pressure release naturally until the float valve drops, and then unlock the lid.
4. Strain the broth and transfer it into a storage container. The broth can be refrigerated for 3–5 days or frozen for 6 months.

Nutrition:

- Calories: 44 kcal
- Fat: 1 g

- Protein: 7 g
- Sodium: 312 mg
- Fiber: 0 g
- Carbohydrates: 0 g
- Sugar: 0 g

64. Chicken Bone Broth With Ginger and Lemon

Preparation Time: 10 minutes

Cooking Time: 90 minutes

Servings: 8

Ingredients:

- Bones from a 3 - 4 pounds chicken
- 8 cups water
- 2 large carrots, cut into chunks
- 2 large stalks celery
- 1 large onion
- 3 fresh rosemary sprigs
- 3 fresh thyme sprigs
- 2 tbsp apple cider vinegar
- 1 tsp kosher salt
- 1-½ inches piece fresh ginger, sliced (peeling not necessary)
- 1 large lemon, cut into fourths

Directions:

1. Put all the ingredients in it and allow it to sit for 30 minutes.
2. Pressure cook and adjust the time to 90 minutes.
3. Set the broth using a fine-mesh strainer and transfer it into a storage container.
4. It can be refrigerated for 5 days or frozen for 5 months.

Nutrition:

- Calories: 44 kcal
- Fat: 1 g
- Protein: 7 g
- Sodium: 312 mg
- Fiber: 0 g
- Carbohydrates: 0 g
- Sugar: 0 g

65. Vegetable Stock

Preparation Time: 10 minutes

Cooking Time: 40 minutes

Servings: 8

Ingredients:

- 2 large carrots
- 1 large onion
- 2 large stalks celery
- 8 oz white mushrooms
- 5 whole cloves garlic
- 2 cups parsley leaves
- 2 bay leaves
- 2 tsp whole black peppercorns
- 2 tsp kosher salt
- 10 cups water

Directions:

1. Place all the ingredients in a pot, secure the lid, and cook for 40 minutes.
2. Set the broth using a fine-mesh strainer and transfer it into a storage container.

Nutrition:

- Calories: 9 kcal
- Fat: 0 g
- Protein: 0 g
- Sodium: 585 mg
- Fiber: 0 g
- Carbohydrates: 2 g
- Sugar: 1 g

66. Chicken Vegetable Soup

Preparation Time: 23 minutes

Cooking Time: 15 minutes

Servings: 8

Ingredients:

- 2 tbsp avocado oil
- 1 small yellow onion, peeled and chopped
- 2 large carrots, peeled and chopped
- 2 large stalks celery, ends removed and sliced
- 3 cloves garlic, minced
- 1 tsp dried thyme
- 1 tsp salt

- 8 cups chicken stock
- 3 boneless, skinless, frozen chicken breasts

Directions:

1. Heat the oil for 1 minute. Add the onion, carrots, and celery and sauté for 8 minutes.
2. Add the garlic, thyme, and salt and sauté for another 30 seconds. Press the Cancel button.
3. Add the stock and frozen chicken breasts to the pot. Secure the lid.
4. Pressure Cook and adjust the time to 6 minutes.
5. Allow cooling into bowls to serve.

Nutrition:

- Calories: 209 kcal
- Fat: 7 g
- Protein: 21 g
- Sodium: 687 mg
- Fiber: 1 g
- Carbohydrates: 12 g
- Sugar: 5 g

67. Carrot Ginger Soup

Preparation Time: 20 minutes

Cooking Time: 21 minutes

Servings: 4

Ingredients:

- 1 tbsp avocado oil
- 1 large yellow onion, peeled and chopped
- 1 pound carrots, peeled and chopped
- 1 tbsp fresh peeled and minced ginger
- 1-½ tsp salt
- 3 cups vegetable broth

Directions:

1. Add the oil to the inner pot, allowing it to heat for 1 minute.
2. Add the onion, carrots, ginger and salt, and sauté for 5 minutes. Press the Cancel button.
3. Add the broth, secure the lid, and adjust the time to 15 minutes.
4. Allow the soup to cool for a few minutes, and then transfer to a large blender. Merge on high until smooth, and then serve.

Nutrition:

- Calories: 99 kcal
- Fat: 4 g
- Protein: 1 g
- Sodium: 1,348 mg
- Fiber: 4 g
- Carbohydrates: 16 g
- Sugar: 7 g

68. Turkey Sweet Potato Hash

Preparation Time: 10 minutes

Cooking Time: 17 minutes

Servings: 4

Ingredients:

- 1-½ tbsp avocado oil
- 1 medium yellow onion, peeled and diced
- 2 cloves garlic, minced
- 1 medium sweet potato, cut into cubes (peeling not necessary)
- ½ lb lean ground turkey
- ½ tsp salt
- 1 tsp Italian seasoning blend

Directions:

1. Attach the oil and allow the oil to heat for 1 minute, and then add the onion and cook until softened, about 5 minutes. Attach the garlic and cook an additional 30 seconds.
2. Add the sweet potato, turkey, salt, and Italian seasoning and cook for another 5 minutes.

Nutrition:

- Calories: 172 kcal
- Fat: 9 g
- Protein: 12 g
- Sodium: 348 mg
- Fiber: 1 g
- Carbohydrates: 10 g
- Sugar: 3 g

69. Turkey Taco Lettuce Boats

Preparation Time: 10 minutes

Cooking Time: 24 minutes

Servings: 4

Ingredients:

- 1 tbsp avocado oil
- 1 medium onion
- 2 large carrots
- 2 medium stalks celery
- 2 cloves garlic, minced
- 1 pound lean ground turkey
- 1 tsp chili powder
- 1 tsp paprika
- 1 tsp cumin
- ½ tsp salt
- ¼ tsp black pepper
- 1 cup chipotle salsa
- 12 large romaine leaves
- 1 medium avocado, peeled, pitted, and sliced

Directions:

1. Add the oil. Set the oil to heat for 1 minute, and then add the onion, carrots, celery, and garlic.
2. Cook until softened, about 5 minutes.
3. Add the turkey and cook until brown for about 3 minutes.
4. Attach the chili powder, paprika, cumin, salt, pepper, and salsa and stir to combine.
5. To serve, set a portion of the taco meat into a romaine lettuce leaf and then top with sliced avocado.

Nutrition:

- Calories: 339 kcal
- Fat: 18 g
- Protein: 27 g
- Sodium: 900 mg
- Fiber: 8 g
- Carbohydrates: 18 g
- Sugar: 8 g

70. Turkey & Greens Meatloaf

Preparation Time: 15 minutes

Cooking Time: 25 minutes

Servings: 4

Ingredients:

- 1 tbsp avocado oil

- 1 small onion, peeled and diced
- 2 Cloves garlic, minced
- 3 cups mixed baby greens, finely chopped
- 1 lb lean ground turkey
- ¼ cup almond flour
- 1 large egg
- ¾ tsp salt
- ½ tsp black pepper

Directions:

1. Add the oil to the inner pot. Press the Sauté button and heat the oil for 1 minute.
2. Attach the onion and sauté for 3 minutes or until softened. Add the garlic and greens and sauté for 1 more minute. Press the Cancel button.
3. Mix the turkey, flour, egg, salt, and pepper in a medium bowl.
4. Add the onion and greens mixture to the turkey mixture and stir to combine.
5. Rinse out the inner pot and then add 2 cups of water.
6. Make an aluminum foil sling by folding a large piece of foil in half and bending the edges upward.
7. Form the turkey mixture into a rectangular loaf and place it on the aluminum foil sling. Place the sling onto the steam rack with handles, and lower it into the inner pot.
8. Carefully remove the meatloaf from the inner pot and allow it to rest for 10 minutes before slicing to serve.

Nutrition:

- Calories: 271 kcal
- Fat: 17 g
- Protein: 25 g
- Sodium: 406 mg
- Fiber: 2 g
- Carbohydrates: 5 g
- Sugar: 1 g

71. Simple Italian Seasoned Turkey Breast

Preparation Time: 10 minutes

Cooking Time: 18 minutes

Servings: 4

Ingredients:

- 1 ½ lb boneless, skinless turkey breast
- 2 tbsp avocado oil, divided
- 1 tsp sweet paprika
- 1 tsp Italian seasoning blend
- ½ tsp kosher salt
- ½ tsp thyme
- ¼ tsp garlic salt
- ¼ tsp black pepper

Directions:

1. Dry the turkey breast with a towel. Cut the turkey breast in half to fit in your Instant Pot.
2. Brush both sides of the turkey breast with 1 tbsp oil.
3. Mix the paprika, Italian seasoning, kosher salt, thyme, garlic, and pepper in a small bowl. Massage this mixture onto both sides of the turkey breast.
4. Press the Sauté button and heat the remaining 1 tbsp oil in the inner pot for 2 minutes.
5. Add the turkey breast and sear it on both sides, about 3 minutes per side. Press the Cancel button.
6. Remove the turkey from the inner pot and place it on a plate.
7. Add 1 cup of water to the inner pot and use a spatula to scrape up any stuck brown bits.
8. Place the steam rack in the pot and the turkey breast on top of it.

Nutrition:

- Calories: 248 kcal
- Fat: 9 g
- Protein: 40 g
- Sodium: 568 mg
- Fiber: 0 g
- Carbohydrates: 0 g
- Sugar: 0 g

72. Spiced Chicken & Vegetables

Preparation Time: 15 minutes

Cooking Time: 15 minutes

Servings: 4

Ingredients:

- 1 tsp thyme, dried
- ¼ tsp ground ginger
- ¼ tsp ground allspice
- 1 tsp kosher salt
- ½ tsp black pepper
- 2 large bone-in chicken breasts
- ½ cup chicken stock
- 2 medium onions, peeled and cut in fourths
- 4 medium carrots

Directions:

1. Mix the thyme, ginger, allspice, salt, and pepper in a small bowl.
2. Use half of the spice mixture to season the chicken breasts.
3. Pour the chicken stock into the inner pot, and then add the chicken breasts.
4. Place the onions and carrots on top of the chicken and sprinkle them with the remaining seasoning blend.
5. Remove the chicken and the vegetables and serve alone or with rice or lentils.

Nutrition:

- Calories: 337 kcal
- Fat: 5 g
- Protein: 56 g
- Sodium: 755 mg
- Fiber: 3 g
- Carbohydrates: 12 g
- Sugar: 5 g

73. Lemon Garlic Turkey Breast

Preparation Time: 10 minutes

Cooking Time: 17 minutes

Servings: 4

Ingredients:

- 1 (1½-pound) boneless, skinless turkey breast
- 2 tbsp avocado oil, divided
- Zest from ½ large lemon
- ½ medium shallot, peeled and minced
- 1 large clove garlic, minced
- ½ tsp kosher salt
- ¼ tsp black pepper

Directions:

1. Dry the turkey breast with a towel.
2. Cut the turkey breast in half to fit in your Instant Pot.
3. Brush both sides of turkey breast with 1 tbsp oil.
4. Mix the lemon zest, shallot, garlic, salt, and pepper in a small bowl. Massage this mixture onto both sides of the turkey breast.
5. Press the Sauté button and heat the remaining 1 tbsp oil in the inner pot for 2 minutes.
6. Add the turkey breast and sear it on both sides, about 3 minutes per side. Press the Cancel button.
7. Remove the turkey from the inner pot and place it on a plate.
8. Add 1 cup of water to the inner pot and use a spatula to scrape up any stuck brown bits.
9. Place the steam rack in the pot and the turkey breast on top of it.
10. Slice and serve.

Nutrition:

- Calories: 250 kcal
- Fat: 9 g
- Protein: 40 g
- Sodium: 445 mg
- Fiber: 0 g
- Carbohydrates: 1 g
- Sugar: 0 g

74. Home-style Chicken & Vegetables

Preparation Time: 5 minutes

Cooking Time: 15 minutes

Servings: 4

Ingredients:

- 2 large bone-in chicken breasts
- 1 tsp kosher salt, divided
- ½ tsp black pepper, divided
- ½ cup chicken stock
- 6 large carrots
- 8 medium whole new potatoes

Directions:

1. Flavor the chicken breasts with ½ tsp salt and ¼ tsp pepper.
2. Pour the stock into the pot.

3. Add chicken breasts and place the carrots and potatoes on top of the chicken.
4. Season with the rest of the salt and pepper.
5. Transfer to the plates to serve and spoon the juices on top.

Nutrition:

- Calories: 398 kcal
- Fat: 5 g
- Protein: 58 g
- Sodium: 822 mg
- Fiber: 5 g

75. Chicken Tenders With Honey Mustard Sauce

Preparation Time: 5 minutes

Cooking Time: 7 minutes

Servings: 4

Ingredients:

- 1 lb chicken tenders
- 1 tbsp fresh thyme leaves
- ½ tsp salt
- ¼ tsp black pepper
- 1 tbsp avocado oil
- 1 cup chicken stock
- ¼ cup Dijon mustard
- ¼ cup raw honey

Directions:

1. Dry the chicken tenders with a towel, and then season them with thyme, salt, and pepper.
2. Attach the oil and let it heat for 2 minutes.
3. Add the chicken tenders and seer them until brown on both sides, about 1 minute per side.
4. Press the Cancel button.
5. Remove the chicken tenders and set them aside.
6. Add the stock to the pot. Use a spoon to scrape up any small bits from the bottom of the pot.
7. Set the steam rack in the inner pot and place the chicken tenders directly on the rack.
8. While the chicken is cooking, set the honey mustard sauce.
9. In a bowl, combine the Dijon mustard and honey and stir to combine.

10. Serve the chicken tenders with the honey mustard sauce.

Nutrition:

- Calories: 223 kcal
- Fat: 5 g
- Protein: 22 g
- Sodium: 778 mg
- Fiber: 0 g
- Carbohydrates: 19 g
- Sugar: 18 g

76. Chicken Breasts With Cabbage & Mushrooms

Preparation Time: 10 minutes

Cooking Time: 18 minutes

Servings: 4

Ingredients:

- 2 tbsp avocado oil
- 1 lb sliced Baby Bella mushrooms
- 1½ tsp salt, divided
- 2 cloves garlic, minced
- 8 cups chopped green cabbage
- 1½ tsp dried thyme
- ½ cup chicken stock
- 1½ lb boneless, skinless chicken breasts

Directions:

1. Add the oil. Allow it to heat for 1 minute.
2. Attach the mushrooms and ¼ tsp salt and sauté until they have cooked down and released their liquid, about 10 minutes.
3. Add the garlic and sauté for another 30 seconds.
4. Press the Cancel button.
5. Add the cabbage, ¼ tsp salt, thyme, and stock to the inner pot and stir to combine.
6. Dry the chicken breasts and sprinkle both sides with the remaining salt.
7. Place on top of the cabbage mixture.
8. Transfer to plates and spoon the juices on top.

Nutrition:

- Calories: 337 kcal
- Fat: 10 g
- Protein: 44 g
- Sodium: 1,023 mg
- Fiber: 4 g
- Carbohydrates: 14 g
- Sugar: 2 g

77. Chicken & Veggie Casserole

Preparation Time: 5 minutes

Cooking Time: 5 minutes

Servings: 4

Ingredients:

- ⅓ cup Dijon mustard
- ⅓ cup organic honey
- 1 tsp dried basil
- ¼ tsp ground turmeric
- 1 tsp dried basil, crushed
- Salt and freshly ground black pepper
- 1¾ lb chicken breast
- 1 cup fresh white mushrooms, sliced
- ½ head broccoli

Directions:

1. Preheat the oven to 350°F. Lightly grease a baking dish.
2. Mix together all ingredients except chicken, mushrooms, and broccoli in a bowl.
3. Set chicken in a prepared baking dish and top with mushroom slices.
4. Place broccoli florets around the chicken evenly.
5. Pour ½ of the honey mixture over chicken and broccoli evenly.
6. Bake for approximately twenty minutes.
7. Cover the chicken with the remaining sauce and bake for approximately 10 minutes.

Nutrition:

- Calories: 248 kcal
- Fat: 9 g
- Protein: 40 g
- Sodium: 568 mg
- Fiber: 0 g

- Carbohydrates: 0 g
- Sugar: 0 g

78. Chicken Meatloaf With Veggies

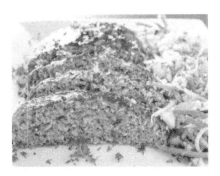

Preparation Time: 20 minutes

Cooking Time: 60 minutes

Servings: 4

Ingredients:

For Meatloaf:

- ½ cup cooked chickpeas
- 2 egg whites
- 2½ tsp poultry seasoning
- Salt and freshly ground black pepper
- 10 oz lean ground chicken
- 1 cup red bell pepper, seeded and minced
- 1 cup celery stalk, minced
- ⅓ cup steel-cut oats
- 1 cup tomato puree, divided
- 2 tbsp dried onion flakes, crushed
- 1 tbsp prepared mustard

For Veggies:

- 2 lbs summer squash, sliced
- 16 oz frozen Brussels sprouts
- 2 tbsp extra-virgin extra virgin olive oil
- Salt and freshly ground black pepper

Directions:

1. Preheat the oven to 350°F.
2. Grease a 9x5-inch loaf pan.
3. Add chickpeas, egg whites, poultry seasoning, salt, and black pepper in a mixer, and pulse till smooth.
4. Transfer the mixture to a large bowl.

5. Add chicken, veggies, oats, ½ cup of tomato puree, and onion flakes and mix till well combined.
6. Transfer the amalgamation into the prepared loaf pan evenly.
7. With both hands, press down the amalgamation slightly.
8. In another bowl, mix mustard and remaining tomato puree.
9. Place the mustard mixture over the loaf pan evenly and bake for approximately 1-1¼ hour or till the desired doneness. Meanwhile, in a big pan of water, arrange a steamer basket.
10. Bring to a boil and set summer time squash I steamer basket.
11. Cover and steam for approximately 10–12 minutes.
12. Drain well and aside.
13. Now, prepare the Brussels sprouts according to the package's directions.
14. Add veggies, oil, salt, and black pepper to a big bowl, and toss to coat well.
15. Serve the meatloaf with veggies.

Nutrition:

- Calories: 337 kcal
- Fat: 5 g
- Protein: 56 g
- Sodium: 755 mg
- Fiber: 3 g
- Carbohydrates: 12 g
- Sugar: 5 g

79.   Roasted Chicken With Veggies & Orange

Preparation Time: 20 minutes

Cooking Time: 60 minutes

Servings: 2

Ingredients:

- 1 tsp ground ginger
- ½ tsp ground cumin
- ½ tsp ground coriander
- 1 tsp paprika
- Salt and freshly ground black pepper
- 1 (3 ½-4-lb) whole chicken
- 1 unpeeled orange, cut into 8 wedges

- 2 medium carrots, peeled and cut into 2-inch pieces
- 2 medium sweet potatoes, peeled and cut into ½-inch wedges
- ½ cup water

Directions:

1. Preheat the oven to 450°F.
2. In a little bowl, mix the spices.
3. Rub the chicken with the spice mixture evenly.
4. Arrange the chicken in a substantial Dutch oven and put orange, carrot, and sweet potato pieces around it.
5. Add water and cover the pan tightly.
6. Roast for around 30 minutes.
7. Uncover and roast for about half an hour.

Nutrition:

- Calories: 216
- Protein: 8.83 g
- Fat: 11.48 g
- Carbs: 21.86 g

80.   Roasted Chicken Drumsticks

Preparation Time: 15 minutes

Cooking Time: 50 minutes

Servings: 2

Ingredients:

- 1 medium onion, chopped
- 1-2 tbsp fresh turmeric, chopped
- 1-2 tbsp fresh ginger, chopped
- 2 lemongrass stalks (bottom third), peeled and chopped
- 1-2 jalapeños, seeded and chopped
- 1 tsp fresh lime zest, grated
- 1 tbsp curry powder
- 1¼ cup unsweetened coconut milk
- 3 tbsp fresh lime juice
- 1 tbsp coconut aminos
- 1 tbsp fish sauce
- 3–4 pounds chicken legs
- Chopped fresh cilantro, for garnish

Directions:

1. Add all ingredients except chicken legs and pulse till smooth in a blender.

2. Transfer the mixture to a large baking dish.
3. Add chicken and coat with marinade generously.
4. Cover and refrigerate to marinate for approximately 12 hours.
5. Take the chicken out of the refrigerator and let it sit at room temperature for about 25 minutes or 1/2 hours before cooking.
6. Preheat the oven to 350°F.
7. Uncover the baking dish and roast for about 50 minutes.

Nutrition:

- Calories: 200
- Carbohydrates: 31 g
- Cholesterol: 93 mg
- Total Fat: 4 g
- Protein: 10 g
- Fiber: 2 g
- Sodium: 288 mg
- Sugar: 10 g

81.   Grilled Chicken Breast

Preparation Time: 15 minutes

Cooking Time: 20 minutes

Servings: 2

Ingredients:

- 2 scallions, chopped
- 1 (1-inch) piece fresh ginger, minced
- 2 minced garlic cloves
- 1 cup fresh pineapple juice
- ¼ cup coconut aminos
- ¼ cup extra-virgin organic olive oil
- 1 tsp ground cinnamon
- 1 tsp ground cumin
- 1 tsp ground turmeric
- Salt, to taste
- 4 skinless, boneless chicken breasts

Directions:

1. In a big Ziploc bag, add all ingredients and seal it.
2. Shake the bag to coat the chicken with marinade well.

3. Refrigerate to marinate for about 20 or so minutes to an hour.
4. Preheat the grill to medium-high heat. Grease the grill grate.
5. Place the chicken pieces on the grill and grill for about 10 min per side.

Nutrition:

- Calories: 200
- Carbohydrates: 31 g
- Cholesterol: 93 mg
- Total Fat: 4 g
- Protein: 10 g
- Fiber: 2 g
- Sodium: 288 mg

82.   Ground Turkey With Veggies

Preparation Time: 15 minutes

Cooking Time: 12 minutes

Servings: 2

Ingredients:

- 1 tbsp sesame oil
- 1 tbsp coconut oil
- 1 lb lean ground turkey
- 2 tbsp fresh ginger, minced
- 2 garlic cloves, minced
- 1 (16-oz) bag vegetable mix (broccoli, carrot, cabbage, kale, and Brussels sprouts)
- ¼ cup coconut aminos
- 2 tbsp balsamic vinegar

Directions:

1. In a big skillet, heat both oils on medium-high heat.
2. Add turkey, ginger, and garlic and cook for approximately 5–6 minutes.
3. Add vegetable mix and cook for approximately 4–5 minutes.
4. Stir in coconut aminos and vinegar and cook for about 1 minute.
5. Serve hot.

Nutrition:

- Calories: 99 kcal
- Fat: 4 g

- Protein: 1 g
- Sodium: 1,348 mg
- Fiber: 4 g
- Carbohydrates: 16 g
- Sugar: 7 g

83. Duck With Bok Choy

Preparation Time: 15 minutes

Cooking Time: 12 minutes

Servings: 6

Ingredients:

- 2 tbsp coconut oil
- 1 onion, sliced thinly
- 2 tsp fresh ginger, grated finely
- 2 garlic cloves, minced
- 1 tbsp fresh orange zest, grated finely
- ¼ cup chicken broth
- ⅔ cup fresh orange juice
- 1 roasted duck, meat picked
- 3 lbs bok choy leaves
- 1 orange, peeled, seeded, and segmented

Directions:

1. In a sizable skillet, melt coconut oil on medium heat. Attach onion, ginger, and garlic, and sauté for around 3 minutes. Add ginger and garlic and sauté for about 1–2 minutes.
2. Stir in orange zest, broth, and orange juice.
3. Add duck meat and cook for around 3 minutes.
4. Transfer the meat pieces to a plate. Add bok choy and cook for about 3–4 minutes.
5. Divide the bok choy mixture into serving plates and top with duck meat.
6. Serve with the garnishing of orange segments.

Nutrition:

- Calories: 290
- Fat: 4 g
- Fiber: 6 g
- Carbs: 8 g
- Protein: 14 g

84. Beef With Mushroom & Broccoli

Preparation Time: 60 minutes

Cooking Time: 12 minutes

Servings: 4

Ingredients:

For Beef Marinade:

- 1 garlic clove, minced
- 1 piece fresh ginger, minced
- Salt and freshly ground black pepper
- 3 tbsp white wine vinegar
- ¾ cup beef broth
- 1 lb flank steak, trimmed and sliced into thin strips

For Vegetables:

- 2 tbsp coconut oil
- 2 garlic cloves
- 3 cups broccoli rabe
- 4-oz shiitake mushrooms
- 8-oz cremini mushrooms

Directions:

1. For marinade in a substantial bowl, mix all ingredients except beef. Add beef and coat with marinade generously. Refrigerate to marinate for around a quarter-hour.
2. In a large skillet, warm oil on medium-high heat.
3. Detach beef from the bowl, reserving the marinade.
4. Attach beef and garlic and cook for about 3–4 minutes or till browned.
5. Add reserved marinade, broccoli, and mushrooms in exactly the same skillet and cook for approximately 3–4 minutes.
6. Set in beef and cook for about 3–4 minutes.

Nutrition:

- Calories: 200
- Carbohydrates: 31 g
- Cholesterol: 93 mg
- Total Fat: 4 g
- Protein: 10 g
- Fiber: 2 g

85. Beef With Zucchini Noodles

Preparation Time: 15 minutes

Cooking Time: 9 minutes

Servings: 4

Ingredients:

- 1 tsp fresh ginger, grated
- 2 medium garlic cloves, minced
- ¼ cup coconut aminos
- 2 tbsp fresh lime juice
- 1½ lb NY strip steak, trimmed and sliced thinly
- 2 medium zucchinis, spiralized with Blade C
- Salt, to taste
- 3 tbsp essential olive oil
- 2 medium scallions, sliced
- 1 tsp red pepper flakes, crushed
- 2 tbsp fresh cilantro, chopped

Directions:

1. Mix the ginger, garlic, coconut aminos, and lime juice in a large bowl. Add beef and coat with marinade generously. Refrigerate to marinate for approximately 10 minutes.
2. Set zucchini noodles over a large paper towel and sprinkle with salt.
3. Keep aside for around 10 minutes.
4. In a large skillet, warm oil on medium-high heat. Attach scallion and red pepper flakes and sauté for about 1 minute. Attach beef with marinade and stir fry for around 3–4 minutes or till browned. Add zucchini and cook for approximately 3–4 minutes.
5. Serve hot.

Nutrition:

- Calories: 1366
- Carbohydrates: 166 g
- Cholesterol: 6 mg
- Total Fat: 67 g
- Protein: 59 g
- Fiber: 41 g

86. Seafood Noodles

Preparation Time: 10 minutes

Cooking Time: 20 minutes

Servings: 2

Ingredients:

- Braised olive oil
- 4 garlic cloves, minced
- 300 g clean squid cut into rings
- 200 g mussel without shell
- 200 g shell-less volley
- 10 clean prawns
- 150 g dried tomatoes
- Salt to taste
- black pepper to taste
- 500 g pre-cooked noodles
- ½ pack watercress
- ½ Lemon Juice
- Parsley to taste

Directions:

1. In olive oil, fix the garlic and add the squid, mussels, prawns, and king prawns, then add the tomatoes and season with salt and pepper and the rest of the ingredients.

Nutrition:

- Calories: 2049
- Protein: 56.21 g
- Fat: 143.36 g
- Carbs: 139.98 g

87. Spicy Pulled Chicken Wraps

Preparation Time: 15 minutes

Cooking Time: 6–8 hours

Servings: 4

Ingredients:

- 1 romaine lettuce head
- 1 ½ tsp ground cumin
- 1 ½ cup low-fat, low-sodium chicken broth
- 1 tsp paprika
- 1 tsp garlic powder
- 1 lb skinless, deboned chicken breasts
- 2 tsp chili powder

Directions:

1. Put all the ingredients except lettuce in a slow cooker and gently stir to combine.
2. Set the slow cooker on Low.
3. Cover and cook for about 6–8 hours.

4. Unsecure the slow cooker and transfer the breasts to a large plate.
5. With a fork, shred the breasts.
6. Serve the shredded beef over lettuce leaves.

Nutrition:

- Calories: 150
- Fat: 3.4 g
- Carbs: 12 g
- Protein: 14 g
- Sugars: 7 g
- Sodium: 900 mg

88. White Bean, Chicken & Apple Cider Chili

Preparation Time: 15 minutes

Cooking Time: 7–8 hours

Servings: 4

Ingredients:

- 3 cups chopped cooked chicken (see Basic "Rotisserie" Chicken)
- 2 (15-oz) cans white navy beans, rinsed well and drained
- 1 medium onion, chopped
- 1 (15-oz) can diced tomatoes
- 3 cups Chicken Bone Broth or store-bought chicken broth
- 1 cup apple cider
- 2 bay leaves
- 1 tbsp extra-virgin olive oil
- 2 tsp garlic powder
- 1 tsp chili powder
- 1 tsp sea salt
- ½ tsp ground cumin
- ¼ tsp ground cinnamon
- Pinch cayenne pepper
- Freshly ground black pepper
- ¼ cup apple cider vinegar

Directions:

1. Using a slow cooker, combine the chicken, beans, onion, tomatoes, broth, cider, bay leaves, olive oil, garlic powder, chili powder, salt, cumin, cinnamon cayenne, then season using black pepper.

2. Cover the cooker and set it to Low.
3. Cook for 7–8 hours.
4. Remove and discard the bay leaves.
5. Stir in the apple cider vinegar until well blended, and serve.

Nutrition:

- Calories: 469
- Total Fat: 8 g
- Total Carbs: 46 g
- Sugar: 13 g
- Fiber: 9 g
- Protein: 51 g
- Sodium: 1,047 mg

89. Beef With Mushroom & Broccoli

Preparation Time: 15 minutes

Cooking Time: 12 minutes

Servings: 4

Ingredients:

For Beef Marinade:

- 1 garlic clove, minced
- 1 (2-inch piece fresh ginger, minced
- Salt, to taste
- Freshly ground black pepper, to taste
- 3 tbsp white wine vinegar
- ¾ cup beef broth
- 1 lb flank steak, trimmed and sliced into thin strips

For Vegetables:

- 2 tbsp coconut oil, divided
- 2 minced garlic cloves
- 3 cups broccoli rabe, chopped
- 4 oz shiitake mushrooms halved
- 8 oz cremini mushrooms, sliced

Directions:

1. For marinade, take a bowl and put together all ingredients except beef. Mix well.
2. Add beef and coat using the marinade.
3. Bring in the fridge to marinate for at least 15 minutes.
4. Using a skillet, warm oil on medium-high heat.

5. Take off beef from the bowl, reserving the marinade.
6. Add beef and garlic and cook for 3–4 minutes or until browned.
7. Using a slotted spoon, put the beef in a bowl.
8. Add the reserved marinade, broccoli, and mushrooms to the same skillet and cook for at least 3–4 minutes.
9. Stir in beef and cook for at least another 3–4 minutes.

Nutrition:

- Calories: 417
- Fat: 10 g
- Carbohydrates: 23 g
- Fiber: 11 g
- Protein: 33 g

9. Serve warm.

Nutrition:

- Calories: 413
- Fat: 24 g
- Carbohydrates: 2 g
- Fiber:1 g
- Protein: 52 g

90.   Mustard Lamb

Preparation Time: 10 minutes

Cooking Time: 35 minutes

Servings: 4

Ingredients:

- 2 (8-rib) lamb racks, patted dry
- ¼ cup Dijon mustard
- 2 tbsp fresh thyme, chopped
- 1 tbsp fresh rosemary, chopped
- Freshly ground black pepper, to taste
- Salt, to taste
- 1 tbsp olive oil

Directions:

1. Preheat an oven to 425°F.
2. In a mixing bowl, combine the mustard, thyme, and rosemary, then mix.
3. Coat the lamb racks with sea salt and pepper.
4. Place a large ovenproof skillet over the medium-high cooking flame and heat the olive oil.
5. Add the lamb rack; stir-cook for about 2 minutes per side, turning once.
6. Take it out from the heat and top with the mustard mix.
7. Bake for 30 minutes or until it cooks well.
8. Remove the lamb racks and cut them into pieces.

Chapter 5. Desserts & Snack

91. Banana Cherry Smoothie

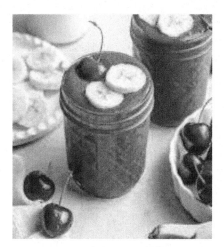

Preparation Time: 5 minutes

Cooking Time: 2 minutes

Servings: 2–3

Ingredients:

- ½ tsp vanilla
- 1 cup cherry
- 2 ½ tbsp chia seeds
- 1 cup unsweetened almond milk
- 1 cup ice cubes
- 1 cup fresh spinach
- 1 banana

Directions:

1. Add all ingredients into the blender and blend until smooth and creamy.
2. Serve and enjoy.

Nutrition:

- Calories: 135
- Fat: 5 g
- Carbohydrates: 20 g
- Sugar: 7 g
- Protein: 4.6 g
- Cholesterol: 0 mg

92. Blueberry & Spinach Smoothie

Preparation Time: 5 minutes

Cooking Time: 2 minutes

Servings: 2–3

Ingredients:

- 2 cups blueberries
- 3 cups fresh spinach, chopped
- ½ cup fresh coriander, chopped
- Juice of 1 lemon
- 1-inch fresh ginger, grated
- 2 cups water

Directions:

1. Put all the ingredients in the blender, and mix for 2 minutes or until smooth.
2. Serve immediately.

Nutrition:

- Calories: 121 |
- Total Carbs: 30.0 g
- Protein: 1.6 g
- Total Fat: 0.6 g
- Sugar: 26.6 g
- Fiber: 2.6 g
- Sodium: 25 mg

93. Matcha Mango Smoothie

Preparation Time: 5 minutes

Cooking Time: 0 minutes

Servings: 2–3

Ingredients:

- 2 cups cubed mango
- 2 tbsp matcha powder
- 2 tsp turmeric powder
- 2 cups almond milk
- 2 tbsp honey
- 1 cup crushed ice

Directions:

1. Combine the mango, matcha, turmeric, almond milk, honey, and ice in a blender. Blend until smooth.
2. Serve immediately.

Nutrition:

- Calories: 285
- Total carbs: 68.0 g
- Protein: 4.0 g
- Total fat: 3.0 g
- Sugar: 63.0 g
- Fiber: 6.0 g
- Sodium: 94 mg

94. Pecan & Lime Cheesecake

Preparation Time: 30 minutes + chilling time

Cooking Time: 0 minutes

Servings: 10

Ingredients:

- 1 cup coconut flakes
- 20 oz mascarpone cheese, room temperature
- 1½ cup pecan meal
- ½ cup xylitol
- 3 tbsp key lime juice

Directions:

1. Combine the pecan meal, ¼ cup of xylitol, and coconut flakes in a mixing bowl. Press the crust into a parchment-lined springform pan. Freeze for 30 minutes.
2. Now, beat the mascarpone cheese with ¼ cup of xylitol with an electric mixer.
3. Beat in the key lime juice; you can add vanilla extract if desired.
4. Spoon the filling onto the prepared crust. Allow it to cool in your refrigerator for about 3 hours. Bon appétit!

Nutrition:

- Calories: 296
- Fat: 20 g
- Carbs: 6 g
- Protein: 21 g
- Fiber: 3.7 g

95. Roasted Potatoes

Preparation Time: 20 minutes

Cooking Time: 30 minutes

Servings: 4

Ingredients:

- 1 red potato wedges
- 1 tbsp rosemary
- 2 garlic cloves
- 1 tbsp olive oil
- ¼ tsp onion powder
- ½ tsp salt
- ½ tsp pepper

Directions:

1. Mix the potato wedges and the rest of the ingredients.
2. Toss to coat the potato wedges and place them on a baking sheet.
3. Bake for 20–25 minutes or until tender.
4. Remove and serve.

Nutrition:

- Calories: 298 kcal
- Fat: 12 g
- Fiber: 2 g
- Carbs: 20 g
- Protein: 5 g

96. Pumpkin Zucchini Muffins

Preparation Time: 10 minutes

Cooking Time: 40 minutes

Servings: 5

Ingredients:

- ½ cup coconut flour
- 1 tsp cinnamon
- ½ tsp baking soda
- ¼ tsp nutmeg
- ¼ tsp mineral salt
- 1 cup homemade pumpkin purée
- 1 ½ cup zucchini, shredded
- 4 organic pasture-raised eggs
- ¼ cup coconut oil, melted
- 3 tbsp honey
- 1 tsp vanilla extract

Directions:

1. Preheat the oven to 350°F. Line a standard muffin tin with a muffin cup.

2. Mix the coconut flour, cinnamon, baking soda, nutmeg, and salt in a large bowl. Whisk together the pumpkin, zucchini, eggs, coconut oil, honey, and vanilla in a separate bowl.
3. Pour the wet ingredients into the dry ingredients and mix to combine.
4. Divide the batter evenly into the muffin cup.
5. Bake for 30–40 minutes or until cooked through and golden on top.

Nutrition:

- Calories: 200 kcal
- Fat: 8 g
- Fiber: 4 g
- Carbs: 8 g
- Protein: 3 g

97.   White Bean Basil Hummus

Preparation Time: 10 minutes

Cooking Time: 0 minutes

Servings: 4

Ingredients:

- 2½ cups white beans, soaked and cooked
- 1 clove garlic
- 2 cups fresh basil
- 2 tbsp homemade tahini
- 2 tbsp lemon juice
- ½ tsp mineral salt
- ¼ cup olive oil, cold-pressed

Directions:

1. In a food processor or high-speed blender, add all the ingredients and blend until smooth. If it is too thick, add a splash of water.
2. Serve with chopped, fresh vegetables (cucumbers, peppers, carrots, or celery).

Nutrition:

- Calories: 298 kcal
- Fat: 12 g
- Fiber: 2 g
- Carbs: 20 g
- Protein: 5 g

98.   Garlic Rosemary Roasted Nuts

Preparation Time: 10 minutes

Cooking Time: 10 minutes

Servings: 4

Ingredients:

- 1 cup almonds
- 1 cup cashews
- 1 cup walnuts
- 2 tbsp coconut oil, melted
- 1 tsp garlic powder
- 2 tsp rosemary, dried, or 1 tbsp fresh rosemary
- ½ tsp mineral salt

Directions:

1. Preheat the oven to 350°F. Line a baking sheet with parchment paper.
2. Add all the ingredients to the baking sheet and toss to coat.
3. Bake for 10 minutes, tossing halfway through.
4. Allow cooling completely before eating.
5. Not suitable for babies.
6. Pack in an airtight container for the perfect packable snack.

Nutrition:

- Calories: 350 kcal
- Fat: 8 g
- Fiber: 2 g
- Carbs: 8 g
- Protein: 26 g

99.   Recipe for Ruby Pears Delight

Preparation Time: 10 minutes

Cooking Time: 10 minutes

Servings: 4

Ingredients:

- 4 pears
- 26 oz grape juice
- 11 oz currant jelly
- 4 garlic cloves
- Juice and zest of 1 lemon
- 4 peppercorns
- 2 rosemary sprigs
- ½ vanilla bean

Directions:

1. Pour the jelly and grape juice into your instant pot and mix with lemon zest and juice
2. In the mix, dip each pear and wrap them in a clean tin foil and place them orderly in the steamer basket of your instant pot
3. Combine peppercorns, rosemary, garlic cloves, and vanilla bean with the juice mixture.
4. Seal the lid and cook at High for 10 minutes.
5. Release the pressure quickly, and carefully open the lid; bring out the pears, remove wrappers and arrange them on plates.
6. Serve when cold with toppings of cooking juice.

Nutrition:

- Calories: 145 kcal
- Fat: 5.6 g
- Fiber: 6 g
- Carbs: 12 g
- Protein: 12 g

100. Mixed Berry & Orange Compote

Preparation Time: 15 minutes

Cooking Time: 15 minutes

Servings: 4

Ingredients:

- ½-lb strawberries
- 1 tbsp orange juice
- ¼ tsp cloves, ground
- ½ cup brown sugar
- 1 vanilla bean
- 1-lb blueberries
- ½-lb blackberries

Directions:

1. Place your berries in the inner pot. Add the sugar and let sit for 15 minutes. Add in the orange juice, ground cloves, and vanilla bean.
2. Secure the lid. Choose the Manual mode and cook for 2 minutes at high pressure. Once cooking is complete, use a natural pressure release for 10 minutes; carefully remove the lid.
3. As your compote cools, it will thicken. Bon appétit!

Nutrition:

- Calories: 224 kcal

- Fat: 0.8 g
- Carbohydrates: 56.3 g
- Protein: 2.1 g
- Sugar: 46.5 g

101. Fig and Homey Buckwheat Pudding

Preparation Time: 10 minutes

Cooking Time: 10 minutes

Servings: 4

Ingredients:

- ½ tsp cinnamon, ground
- ½ cup figs, dried and chopped
- ⅓ cup honey
- 1 tsp pure vanilla extract
- 3½ cup milk
- ½ tsp pure almond extract
- 1½ cup buckwheat

Directions:

1. Add all the above ingredients to your Instant Pot.
2. Secure the lid. Choose the "Multigrain" mode and cook for 10 minutes under high pressure. Once cooking is complete, use a natural pressure release; carefully remove the lid.
3. Serve topped with fresh fruits, nuts, or whipped topping. Bon appétit!

Nutrition:

- Calories: 320 kcal
- Fat: 7.5 g
- Carbohydrates: 57.7 g
- Protein: 9.5 g
- Sugar: 43.2 g

102. Zingy Blueberry Sauce

Preparation Time: 5 minutes

Cooking Time: 20 minutes

Servings: 10

Ingredients:

- ¼ cup fresh lemon juice

- 1 lb sugar, granulated
- 1 tbsp lemon zest, freshly grated
- ½ tsp vanilla extract
- 2 lbs fresh blueberries

Directions:

1. Place the blueberries, sugar, and vanilla in the inner pot of your Instant Pot.
2. Secure the lid. Choose the "Manual" mode and cook for 2 minutes at high pressure. Once cooking is complete, use a natural pressure release for 15 minutes; carefully remove the lid.
3. Stir in the lemon zest and juice. Puree in a food processor; then strain and push the mixture through a sieve before storing. Enjoy!

Nutrition:

- Calories: 230 kcal
- Fat: 0.3 g
- Carbohydrates: 59 g
- Protein: 0.7 g
- Sugar: 53.6 g

2. Add the remaining ingredients in the order listed above. Divide the batter among 3 ramekins.
3. Add 1 cup of water and a metal trivet to the Instant Pot.
4. Cover ramekins with foil and lower them onto the trivet.
5. Secure the lid and select Manual mode.
6. Cook at high pressure for 12 minutes. Once cooking is complete, use a quick release; carefully remove the lid.
7. Transfer the ramekins to a wire rack and allow them to cool slightly before serving.
8. Enjoy!

Nutrition:

- Calories: 304 kcal
- Fat: 18.9 g
- Carbohydrates: 23.8 g
- Protein: 10 g
- Sugar: 21.1 g

103. Chocolate Almond Custard

Preparation Time: 10 minutes

Cooking Time: 15 minutes

Servings: 3

Ingredients:

- 3 chocolate cookies, chunks
- A pinch salt
- ¼ tsp cardamom, ground
- 3 tbsp honey
- ¼ tsp nutmeg, freshly grated
- 2 tbsp butter
- 3 tbsp whole milk
- 1 cup almond flour
- 3 eggs
- 1 tsp pure vanilla extract

Directions:

1. In a mixing bowl, beat the eggs with butter. Now, add the milk and continue mixing until well combined.

104. Jasmine Rice Pudding With Cranberries

Preparation Time: 5 minutes

Cooking Time: 15 minutes

Servings: 4

Ingredients:

- 1 cup apple juice
- 1 heaping tbsp honey
- ⅓ cup sugar, granulated
- 1½ cup jasmine rice
- 1 cup water
- ¼ tsp cinnamon, ground
- ¼ tsp cloves, ground
- ⅓ tsp cardamom, ground
- 1 tsp vanilla extract
- 3 eggs, well-beaten
- ½ cup cranberries

Directions:

1. Thoroughly combine the apple juice, honey, sugar, jasmine rice, water, and spices in the inner pot of your Instant Pot.
2. Secure the lid. Choose the Manual mode and cook for 4 minutes at high pressure. Once cooking is complete, use a natural pressure release for 5 minutes; carefully remove the lid.
3. Press the Sauté button and fold in the eggs. Cook on Less mode until heated through.
4. Ladle into individual bowls and top with dried cranberries. Enjoy!

Nutrition:

- Calories: 402 kcal
- Fat:3.6 g
- Carbs:81.1 g
- Protein: 8.9 g
- Sugar: 22.3 g
- Fiber: 2.2 g

105. Vanilla Ice Cream

Preparation Time: 10 minutes

Cooking Time: 0 minutes

Servings: 8

Ingredients:

- 3 cups full-fat coconut milk
- ⅓ cup maple syrup
- 2 tsp vanilla extract
- ¼ tsp salt

Directions:

1. Whisk together the coconut milk, maple syrup, vanilla, and salt in a large bowl. Alternately, use a blender to combine. 2. If using an ice cream maker, freeze according to the manufacturers. Transfer the ice cream to a sealed container and store it in the freezer.
2. You can also freeze some of the mixture in ice cube trays to add to smoothies.

Nutrition:

- Calories: 296
- Fat: 24 g
- Protein: 2 g
- Carbs: 18 g
- Fiber: 0 g
- Sugar: 14 g
- Sodium: 129 mg

106. Rich Carob Sheet Cake

Preparation Time: 10 minutes

Cooking Time: 40 minutes

Servings: 12

Ingredients:

- 1 cup melted coconut oil, plus more for greasing the baking dish
- 10 eggs
- 1 cup pure maple syrup
- 2 tsp pure vanilla extract
- ¾ cup coconut flour
- ½ cup carob powder
- 1 tsp baking soda
- ⅛ tsp sea salt

Directions:

1. Preheat the oven to 350ºF (180ºC).
2. Lightly grease a 9-by-13-inch baking dish with coconut oil and set it aside.

3. In a large bowl, beat or whisk the eggs until frothy.
4. Add the remaining 1 cup of coconut oil, maple syrup, and vanilla. Beat or whisk until well blended.
5. In a small bowl, stir together the coconut flour, carob powder, baking soda, and sea salt. Add the dry ingredients to the wet ingredients and blend until smooth. Pour the batter into the prepared dish.
6. Bake for about 40 minutes or until a knife inserted in the center comes out clean.
7. Remove the cake from the oven and let it cool on a wire rack.
8. Serve with fruit or topped with whipped coconut cream, if desired.

Nutrition:

- Calories: 312
- Fat: 25 g
- Protein: 6 g
- Carbs: 21 g
- Fiber: 2 g
- Sugar: 16 g
- Sodium: 74 mg

107. Banana "Nice" Cream

Preparation Time: 5 minutes

Cooking Time: 0 minutes

Servings: 4

Ingredients:

- 4 frozen, diced bananas

Directions:

1. In a food processor or blender, blend the bananas for 3–5 minutes until they reach a whipped, creamy consistency. Depending on how frozen the bananas are, it may take a bit longer.
2. Serve immediately.

Nutrition:

- Calories: 112
- Fat: 0 g
- Protein: 1 g
- Carbs: 29 g
- Fiber: 3 g
- Sugar: 14 g
- Sodium: 1 mg

108. Key Lime Pie Pots De Crème

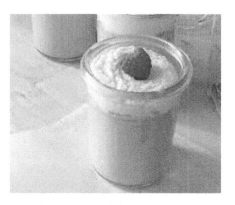

Preparation Time: 30 minutes

Cooking Time: 15 minutes

Servings: 3

Ingredients:

Filling:

- 1 (13½-oz / 383-g) can full-fat coconut milk
- 2 tsp pure vanilla extract
- 1 tsp grated lime zest
- Juice of 2 limes
- 20 drops liquid stevia
- Pinch of fine Himalayan salt
- 1 stalk lemongrass, cut into 3 pieces
- 1 heaping tbsp unflavored grass-fed beef gelatin

Hemp Seed Crumble:

- ½ cup shelled hemp seeds (aka hemp hearts)
- 1 tsp raw honey
- 1 tsp grated lime zest
- Pinch of fine Himalayan salt

Directions:

Make the Filling:

1. Combine the coconut milk, vanilla extract, lime zest, lime juice, stevia, salt, and lemongrass in a small saucepan over medium-low heat.
2. Cook, occasionally stirring, for 5 minutes or until the milk begins to steam. It will become aromatic and begin to bubble a little on the edges.
3. Use tongs or a slotted spoon to remove the pieces of lemongrass.
4. As you whisk the coconut milk mixture, sprinkle in the gelatin until it is fully dissolved. Remove the pan from the heat.
5. Pour the mixture through a fine-mesh sieve into 3 4-oz (113-g) ramekins.
6. Refrigerate for 30–45 minutes until set.
7. Place the ramekins in the coldest part of the refrigerator, usually the back of the top shelf.

Make the Hemp Seed Crumble:

8. Combine the hemp seeds, honey, lime zest, and salt in a small skillet over medium heat. Cook, stirring slowly, for 5–6 minutes. The seeds will begin to toast, and the mixture will smell sweet and popcorn-like. Remove the pan from the heat when most of the seeds are browned.
9. Use a spoon to flatten the mixture and set it under a fan to cool while the pots de crème finish setting.
10. When the pots de crème are ready, remove them from the refrigerator.
11. Use a spoon to break up the candied hemp seeds and sprinkle them over the pots de crème for a crunchy, toasty, sweet crust.
12. These are best enjoyed right away. The creamy pots will turn full-on firm if they set any longer.

Nutrition:

Calories: 368 | fat: 33 g | protein: 11 g | carbs: 19 g | fiber: 6 g | sugar: 11 g | sodium: 238 mg

109. Apricot Biscotti

Preparation Time: 10 minutes

Cooking Time: 40 minutes

Servings: 4–6

Ingredients:

- ¾ cup bran flour (whole wheat)
- ¾ cup common flour (white)
- ¼ cup brown sugar, very compact
- 1 tsp baking powder
- 2 eggs, lightly beaten
- 2 tbsp 1 percent low-fat milk
- 2 tbsp canola oil
- 2 tbsp dark honey
- ½ tsp almond extract
- ⅔ cup chopped dried apricots
- ¼ cup large, chopped almonds

Directions:

1. Warm the oven to 350°F (175°C).
2. Place the flour, brown sugar, and baking powder in a large bowl.
3. Beat until mixed. Add eggs, milk, canola oil, honey, and almond extract.
4. Set with a wooden spoon until the dough begins to integrate. Add almonds and chopped apricots. With floured hands, mix the dough until the ingredients are well integrated.
5. Place the dough on a large sheet of plastic wrap and form a crushed roll 12 inches (30 cm) long, 3 inches (7.5 cm) wide, and about 1 inch (2.5 cm) by hand.
6. High Lift the plastic wrap and invert the dough into a non-stick baking sheet. Bake for 25–30 minutes, until lightly browned.
7. Transfer it to another baking sheet and let it cool for 10 minutes. Leave the oven at 350°F (175°C).
8. Place the cold dough on a cutting board and cut transversely into 24 ½ inches (1 cm) wide portions with a serrated knife. Place the pieces with the cut down on the baking sheet.
9. Bake again for 15–20 minutes, until crispy. Go to a rack and let cool completely.
10. Store in an airtight container.

Nutrition:

- Calories: 75
- Total Fat: 2 g
- Cholesterol: 15 mg
- Sodium: 17 mg
- Total carbohydrate: 12 g
- Dietary fiber: 1 g
- Total sugars: 6 g
- Added sugars: 2 g
- Protein: 2 g

110. Chocolate Mascarpone

Preparation Time: 10 minutes

Cooking Time: 40 minutes

Servings: 4–6

Ingredients:

- 250ml fondant cream (well chilled)
- 250 g Mascarpone cheese
- 200 g Dark chocolate
- 4 tbsp powdered sugar

Directions:

1. Applying cream, we dissolve chocolate in a water bath, i.e., place the chocolate in a glass bowl. Set the bowl on a pot with boiling water—so that the bottom of the bowl does not touch the water.
2. Leave the melted chocolate to cool (until it is not hot, only slightly warm). Whip cream. Mix mascarpone cheese with a mixer with powdered sugar. Without stopping the mixer, add chocolate to the cheese (gently pour in a small stream). Mix until smooth.
3. Add whipped cream to the chocolate mass. Then mix manually or with a mixer at low speed until we get a uniform, creamy, thick consistency.
4. Apply the cream to the cup using the sleeve to decorate the cakes to get a nice-looking dessert. We store the ready cream in the fridge.

Nutrition:

- Calories: 591
- Protein: 11.03 g
- Fat: 53.8 g
- Carbs: 26.58 g

111. Almond Ricotta Spread

Preparation Time: 10 minutes

Cooking Time: 35 minutes

Servings: 5

Ingredients:

- 200 gr. raw and unsalted almonds
- 100 gr. raw and unsalted cashews
- 2 tbsp lemon juice
- Sea salt at ease
- 1 tbsp of yeast in "Titan"
- Black pepper to taste
- Fresh herbs to taste (rosemary, parsley, dill, sage, thyme, coriander)

Directions:

1. Soak the nuts.
2. The next day, strain the nuts and process them with lemon juice, salt, flaked yeast (or very fine-grated "Viol life" cheese), and pepper until a thick cream is formed.
3. Turn the processor on and off if necessary, and stir well so that everything is well integrated.
4. Some water can be added, but not in excess, to prevent the dip from becoming too liquid. It should have the consistency of the traditional "pillory."
5. Rectify the salt and pepper again and add fresh herbs on top.

Nutrition:

- Calories: 591
- Protein: 11.03 g
- Fat: 53.8 g
- Carbs: 26.58 g

112. Berry Compote

Preparation Time: 10 minutes

Cooking Time: 5 minutes

Servings: 8

Ingredients:

- 1 cup blueberries
- 2 cups strawberries, sliced
- 2 tbsp lemon juice
- ¾ cup sugar
- 1 tbsp cornstarch
- 1 tbsp water

Directions:

1. In the Instant Pot, mix the blueberries with lemon juice and sugar, stir, cover, and cook on the Manual setting for 3 minutes.

2. Mix the cornstarch with water in a bowl, stir well, and add to the Instant Pot. Stir, set the Instant Pot on Sauté mode, and cook compote for 2 minutes.
3. Divide into jars and keep in the refrigerator until you serve it.

Nutrition:

- Calories: 260 kcal
- Fat: 13 g
- Fiber: 3 g
- Carbs: 23 g
- Protein: 3 g

113. Fruit Cobbler

Preparation Time: 10 minutes

Cooking Time: 12 minutes

Servings: 4

Ingredients:

- 3 apples, cored and cut into chunks
- 2 pears, cored and cut into chunks
- 1½ cup hot water
- ¼ cup honey
- 1 cup steel-cut oats
- 1 tsp cinnamon, ground
- Ice cream, for serving

Directions:

1. Put the apples and pears into the Instant Pot and mix with hot water, honey, oats, and cinnamon.
2. Stir, cover, and cook on the Manual setting for 12 minutes.
3. Release the pressure naturally, transfer the cobbler to a plate and serve.

Nutrition:

- Calories: 170 kcal
- Fat: 4 g
- Carbs: 10 g
- Fiber: 2.4 g
- Protein: 3 g
- Sugar: 7 g

114. Stuffed Peaches

Preparation Time: 10 minutes

Cooking Time: 4 minutes

Servings: 6

Ingredients:

- 6 peaches, pits, and flesh removed
- Salt
- ¼ cup coconut flour
- ¼ cup maple syrup
- 2 tbsp coconut butter
- ½ tsp cinnamon, ground
- 1 tsp almond extract
- 1 cup water

Directions:

1. Mix the flour with the salt, syrup, butter, cinnamon, and half of the almond extract in a bowl and stir well.
2. Fill the peaches with this mix, place them in the steamer basket of the Instant Pot, add the water and the rest of the almond extract to the Instant Pot, cover, and cook on the Steam setting for 4 minutes.
3. Release the pressure, divide the stuffed peaches on serving plates, and serve warm.

Nutrition:

- Calories: 160 kcal
- Fat: 6.7 g
- Carbs: 12 g
- Fiber: 3 g
- Sugar: 11 g
- Protein: 4 g

115. Peach Compote

Preparation Time: 10 minutes

Cooking Time: 3 minutes

Servings: 6

Ingredients:

- 8 peaches, pitted and chopped
- 6 tbsp sugar
- 1 tsp cinnamon, ground
- 1 tsp vanilla extract

- 1 vanilla bean, scraped
- 2 tbsp Grape Nuts cereal

Directions:

1. Put the peaches into the Instant Pot and mix with the sugar, cinnamon, vanilla bean, and vanilla extract.
2. Stir well, cover the Instant Pot, and cook on the Manual setting for 3 minutes.
3. Release the pressure for 10 minutes, add the cereal, stir well, transfer the compote to bowls, and serve.

Nutrition:

- Calories: 100 kcal
- Fat: 2 g
- Carbs: 11 g
- Fiber: 1 g
- Sugar: 10 g
- Protein: 1 g

116.   Chocolate Pudding

Preparation Time: 10 minutes

Cooking Time: 20 minutes

Servings: 4

Ingredients:

- 6 oz bittersweet chocolate, chopped
- ½ cup milk
- 1½ cup heavy cream
- 5 egg yolks
- ⅓ cup brown sugar
- 2 tsp vanilla extract
- 1½ cup water
- ¼ tsp cardamom
- Salt
- Crème fraiche, for serving
- Chocolate shavings, for serving

Directions:

1. Put the cream and milk in a pot, bring to a simmer over medium heat, take off the heat, add the chocolate and whisk well.
2. In a bowl, mix the egg yolks with the vanilla, sugar, cardamom, and a pinch of salt, stir, strain, and mix with the chocolate mixture.

3. Pour this into a soufflé dish, cover with aluminum foil, place in the steamer basket of the Instant Pot, add water to the Instant Pot, cover, cook on Manual for 18 minutes, and release the pressure naturally.
4. Take the pudding out of the Instant Pot, set aside to cool down, and keep it in the refrigerator for 3 hours before serving with crème Fraiche and chocolate shavings on top.

Nutrition:

- Calories: 200 kcal
- Fat: 3 g
- Fiber: 1 g
- Carbs: 20 g
- Protein: 14 g

117.   Refreshing Curd

Preparation Time: 10 minutes

Cooking Time: 5 minutes

Servings: 4

Ingredients:

- 3 tbsp stevia
- 12 oz raspberries
- 2 egg yolks
- 2 tbsp lemon juice
- 2 tbsp ghee

Directions:

1. Put raspberries in your instant pot, add stevia and lemon juice, stir, cover, and cook on High for 2 minutes.
2. Strain this into a bowl, add egg yolks, stir well, and return to your pot.
3. Set the pot on Simmer mode, cook for 2 minutes, add ghee, stir well, transfer to a container and serve cold.
4. Enjoy!

Nutrition:

- Calories: 132 kcal
- Fat: 1 g
- Fiber: 0 g
- Carbohydrates: 2 g
- Protein: 4 g

118. Honey Stewed Apples

Preparation Time: 5 minutes

Cooking Time: 5 minutes

Servings: 4

Ingredients:

- 2 tbsp honey
- 1 tsp cinnamon, ground
- ½ tsp cloves, ground
- 4 apples

Directions:

1. Add all ingredients to the inner pot. Now, pour in ⅓ cup of water.
2. Secure the lid. Choose the Manual mode and cook for 2 minutes at high pressure. Once cooking is complete, use a quick pressure release; carefully remove the lid.
3. Serve in individual bowls.
4. Bon appétit!

Nutrition:

- Calories: 128 kcal
- Fat: 0.3 g
- Carbohydrates: 34.3 g
- Protein: 0.5 g
- Sugar: 27.5 g

119. Baklava With Lemon Honey Syrup

Preparation Time: 10 minutes

Cooking Time: 0 minutes

Servings: 3

Ingredients:

- 400 g of filo pastry
- 300 g of walnuts
- 250 g of pistachios
- 200 g of butter
- 200 g of sugar
- A tbsp of lemon juice
- 2 tbsp of honey
- 300 ml of water

Directions:

1. Melt the butter in a saucepan and let it cool while chopping the pistachios and almonds together with 2 tablespoons of sugar.
2. Butter the pan, then spread the first sheet of phyllo dough, brush it with the melted butter and place a second and a third on it, still buttering.
3. After the third layer, place chopped walnuts and pistachios and start the process again: for every 3 sheets of buttered pasta, insert a layer of walnuts and pistachios until you finish with the filo pastry.
4. Bake at 180º for 15 minutes.
5. Meanwhile, prepare the syrup and bring the sugar, water, lemon juice, and honey to a boil (over medium heat, stirring constantly).
6. Once cooked, sprinkle the syrup baklava, and let it cool.
7. Serve cut into diamonds and covered with chopped walnuts and pistachios.

Nutrition:

- Calories: 591
- Protein: 11.03 g
- Fat: 53.8 g
- Carbs: 26.58 g

120. Greek Butter Cookies

Preparation Time: 5–10 minutes

Cooking Time: 5 minutes

Servings: 4

Ingredients:

- 150 g raw almonds
- 155 g soft butter (at room temperature)
- 70 g caster sugar
- 2 egg yolks
- 300 g flour 00
- ½ tsp baking powder
- Icing sugar to taste
- 20 whole cloves

Directions:

1. Bring a saucepan to boil with water. When the water boils, add the almonds, cook for 10 minutes, and then drain on a sheet of absorbent paper. Remove the almond skin.
2. Light the oven to 200°C, cover a baking sheet with baking paper, and toast the almonds. When they are well toasted, let them cool. Once cold, whisk it with a chopper. Do not reduce them to flour, but get a fine grain.
3. Whip the butter with the sugar, helping yourself with the electric whisk until you get froth. Add the egg yolks and mix with the whisk until all the ingredients are mixed. Sift the flour and baking powder.
4. Attach the flour, baking powder, and chopped almonds to the dough. Start kneading in the bowl, then move to a table and knead; it takes patience before the dough becomes compact. As soon as you get compact dough, wrap it in plastic wrap and let it rest in the fridge for an hour.
5. As soon as this time has elapsed, preheat the oven to 180°C and cover a baking sheet with baking paper. Set balls about the size of a walnut and place them on the baking tray, placing them at 2 cm from each other.
6. Press the center of each ball with the fingertips to obtain a small furrow and until golden brown. When baked, put a clove in the center of each cookie.
7. Let them cool, and then sprinkle with plenty of icing sugar.

Nutrition:

- Calories: 42
- Protein: 3.13 g
- Fat: 1.68 g
- Carbs: 4.77 g

121.   Cocoa Muffins With Coffee

Preparation Time: 10 minutes

Cooking Time: 20 minutes

Servings: 2

Ingredients:

- ½ hour soft butter
- 1 egg
- 1 tsp sugar
- 1 tsp vanilla
- 1 -½ tsp flour
- 1 tsp baking soda
- Salt
- ½ tsp cocoa
- ½ tsp yogurt
- ⅓ tsp strong coffee

Directions:

1. Beat the butter with the sugar, and add the egg and vanilla.
2. Mix flour, baking soda, and salt, cocoa separately.
3. Add the dry ingredients of the parts together with the yogurt and the coffee parts to the egg mixture.
4. Warm the oven to 180°C, fill the muffin cups with ⅔ of the mixture, and bake for 20–25 minutes or until ready.
5. For the glaze, I experimented and made it with liquid pastry cream / about ¾ cup of tea / and a packet of 1 kg powdered sugar (I didn't get the whole packet). The mixture should be thick.
6. Enjoy!!

Nutrition:

- Calories: 95
- Fat: 3.3 g
- Fiber: 1.3 g
- Carbs: 10.1 g
- Protein: 6.4 g

122.   Low Carb Nougat Whims

Preparation Time: 10 minutes

Cooking Time: 40 minutes

Servings: 4–6

Ingredients:

- 210 g dark chocolate with a minimum of 70% cocoa solids
- 125 ml (110 g) coconut oil, divided
- 400 g coconut milk, only the solid part
- 8 tbsp peanut butter or other nut butter you like
- 1 tbsp (5 g) cocoa powder
- 1 tsp vanilla extract

Directions:

1. Dissolve half of the chocolate in a water bath or microwave over low heat. Add a quarter of coconut oil and mix well.
2. Pour into a greased mold and coated with baking paper (approximately 13 x 20 inches, if you make 40) and let cool in the refrigerator or freezer.
3. Carefully heat the solid part of the coconut milk (canned) in a different pan. Let it simmer for a few minutes.
4. Add half of the coconut oil, nut butter, cocoa powder, and vanilla while stirring. Make a smooth mixture. If the dough separates, use a hand blender and press several times to make it uniform.
5. Detach from heat and pour over the chocolate. Set the pan to the refrigerator or freezer to cool again while the rest of the chocolate melts, as in step 1.
6. Attach the remaining coconut oil to the chocolate and mix. Spread it in a layer over the cold nougat. Replace in the refrigerator and let stand for at least an hour, preferably longer.
7. Cut into 30–40 small pieces. Set in an airtight container in the refrigerator or freezer. The nougat is best served slightly cold.

Nutrition:

- Calories: 288
- Fat: 12 g
- Sat Fat: 1 g
- Carbohydrates: 41 g
- Fiber: 5 g
- Protein: 6 g
- Sodium: 125 mg

123. Raspberry Feast Meringue With Cream Diplomat

Preparation Time: 10 minutes

Cooking Time: 60 minutes

Servings: 4

Ingredients:

- 2 egg whites
- ½ cup caster sugar
- ¼ tsp vanilla extract
- ¼ cup crumbled barley sugar
- 1 cup frozen raspberries
- ¼ cup water
- 2 tbsp Raspberry Jell-O Powder with No Added Sugar
- 1½ cup Cool Whip
- 1 bowl fresh raspberries

Directions:

1. Preheat the oven to 350°F (175°C) to make the meringue, and line a baking sheet with parchment paper.
2. Whisk egg whites in a blender or bowl until the foam is obtained. Gently add the sugar while whisking until you get firm, shiny picks. Stir in vanilla extract and crumbled barley sugar.
3. Shape the meringues on the coated cookie sheet and place them in the preheated oven. Turn off the oven and wait 2 hours. Do not open the oven. Once the meringues are dry, break them into small bites.
4. To make the mousse, put frozen raspberries and water in a small saucepan. Heat until raspberries melt and are tender. Put these raspberries in a blender. Add the Jell-O powder and mix. Once the raspberries have completely cooled, incorporate the Cool Whip.
5. To shape the raspberry, place in balloon glasses for individual portions or in a large cake pan first a layer of raspberry mousse, then a layer of meringue, then fresh raspberries. Repeat the layers. Refrigerate for a few hours before serving.

Nutrition:

- Calories: 99 kcal
- Fat: 4 g
- Protein: 1 g
- Sodium: 1,348 mg
- Fiber: 4 g
- Carbohydrates: 16 g
- Sugar: 7 g

124. Cheesecake Mousse With Raspberries

Preparation Time: 10 minutes

Cooking Time: 40 minutes

Servings: 4–6

Ingredients:

- 1 cup light lemonade filling
- 1 can (8 oz) cream cheese at room temperature
- ¾ cup Splenda no-calorie sweetener pellets
- 1 tbsp lemon zest
- 1 tbsp vanilla extract
- 1 cup fresh or frozen raspberries

Directions:

1. Beat the cream cheese until it is sparkling; add ½ cup Splenda Granules and mix until melted. Stir in lemon zest and vanilla.
2. Reserve some raspberries for decoration. Set the rest of the raspberries with a fork and mix them with ¼ cup Splenda pellets until they are melted.
3. Lightly add the lump and cheese filling, and then gently but quickly add crushed raspberries.
4. Share this mousse in 6 ramekins with a spoon and keep in the refrigerator until tasting. Garnish mousses with reserved raspberries and with fresh mint.

Nutrition:

- Calories: 734
- Carbohydrates: 37 g
- Cholesterol: 115 mg
- Total Fat: 54 g
- Protein: 25 g

125.   Almond Meringue Cookies

Preparation Time: 10 minutes

Cooking Time: 30 minutes

Servings: 2

Ingredients:

- 2 egg whites or 4 tbsp pasteurized egg whites
- 1 tbsp tartar cream
- ½ tsp
- ½ tsp almond extract vanilla extract
- ½ cup white sugar

Directions:

1. Preheat the oven to 300°F.
2. Set the egg whites with the cream of tartar until the volume has doubled. Add other ingredients and whip until peaks form.
3. Using 2 tsp, drop a spoonful of meringue onto parchment paper with the back of the other spoon.
4. Bake at 300°F for about 25 minutes or until the meringues are crisp. Place in an airtight container.

Nutrition:

- Calories: 198
- Fat: 7.7 g
- Fiber: 3.5 g
- Carbs: 27.9 g
- Protein: 4.7 g

126.   Chai Spice Baked Apples

Preparation Time: 15 minutes

Cooking Time: 2 to 3 hours

Servings: Makes 5 apples

Ingredients:

- 5 apples
- ½ cup water
- ½ cup crushed pecans (optional)
- ¼ cup melted coconut oil
- 1 tsp ground cinnamon
- ½ tsp ground ginger
- ¼ tsp ground cardamom
- ¼ tsp ground cloves

Directions:

1. Core each apple, and peel off a thin strip from the top of each.
2. Add the water to the slow cooker.
3. Gently place each apple upright along the bottom.
4. In a small bowl, stir together the pecans (if using), coconut oil, cinnamon, ginger, cardamom, and cloves. Drizzle the mixture over the tops of the apples.
5. Cover the cooker and set it to high.
6. Cook for 2–3 hours, until the apples soften, and serve.

Nutrition:

- Calories: 217
- Fat: 12 g
- Protein: 0 g
- Carbs: 30 g
- Fiber: 6 g
- Sugar: 20 g
- Sodium: 0 mg

127. Maple-Glazed Pears With Hazelnuts

Preparation Time: 10 minutes

Cooking Time: 20 minutes

Servings: 4

Ingredients:

- 4 pears, peeled, cored, and quartered lengthwise
- 1 cup apple juice
- ½ cup pure maple syrup
- 1 tbsp grated fresh ginger
- ¼ cup chopped hazelnuts

Directions:

1. Combine the pears and apple juice in a large pot over medium-high heat. Bring to a simmer and reduce the heat to medium-low.
2. Cover and simmer for 15–20 minutes until the pears soften. While the pears poach, combine the maple syrup and ginger in a small saucepan over medium-high heat. Bring to a simmer, stirring. Remove the pan from the heat and let it rest.
3. Using a slotted spoon, remove the pears from the poaching liquid and brush with the maple syrup. Serve topped with hazelnuts.

Nutrition:

- Calories: 286
- Fat: 3 g
- Protein: 2 g
- Carbs: 67 g
- Fiber: 7 g
- Sugar: 50 g
- Sodium: 9 mg

128. Gluten-Free Oat & Fruit Bars

Preparation Time: 15 minutes

Cooking Time: 40–45 minutes

Servings: Makes 16 bars

Ingredients:

- Cooking spray
- ½ cup maple syrup
- ½ cup almond or sunflower butter
- 2 medium ripe bananas, mashed
- ⅓ cup dried cranberries
- 1½ cup old-fashioned rolled oats
- ½ cup shredded coconut
- ¼ cup oat flour
- ¼ cup ground flaxseed
- 1 tsp vanilla extract
- ½ tsp ground cinnamon
- ¼ tsp ground cloves

Directions:

1. Preheat the oven to 400°F (205°C).
2. Line an 8-by-8-inch square pan with parchment paper or aluminum foil, and coat the lined pan with cooking spray.
3. Mix the maple syrup, almond butter, and bananas in a medium bowl. Mix until well blended.
4. Add the cranberries, oats, coconut, oat flour, flaxseed, vanilla, cinnamon, and cloves. Mix well.
5. Spoon the mixture into the prepared pan; the mixture will be thick and sticky. Use an oiled spatula to spread the mixture evenly.
6. Place the pan in the preheated oven and bake for 40–45 minutes, until the top is dry and a toothpick inserted in the middle comes clean. Cool completely before cutting into bars.

Nutrition:

- Calories: 144
- Fat: 7 g
- Protein: 3 g
- Carbs: 19 g
- Fiber: 2 g
- Sugar: 8 g
- Sodium: 3 mg

129. Orange & Almond Cupcakes

Preparation Time: 5 minutes

Cooking Time: 20 minutes

Servings: 9

Ingredients:

Cupcakes:

- 1 orange extract
- 2 tbsp olive oil
- 2 tbsp ghee, at room temperature
- 3 eggs, beaten
- 2 oz Greek yogurt
- 2 cups cake flour
- A pinch salt
- 1 tbsp orange rind, grated
- ½ cup brown sugar
- ½ cup almonds, chopped

Cream cheese frosting:

- 2 oz cream cheese
- 1 tbsp whipping cream
- ½ cup butter, at room temperature
- 1 ½ cup confectioners' sugar, sifted
- ⅓ tsp vanilla
- A pinch salt

Directions:

1. Mix the orange extract, olive oil, ghee, eggs, and Greek yogurt until well combined.
2. Thoroughly combine the cake flour, salt, orange rind, and brown sugar in a separate mixing bowl. Add the egg/yogurt mixture to the flour mixture. Stir in the chopped almonds and mix again.
3. Place parchment baking liners on the bottom of a muffin tin. Pour the batter into the muffin tin.
4. Place 1 cup of water and a metal trivet in the inner pot of your Instant Pot. Lower the prepared muffin tin onto the trivet.
5. Secure the lid. Choose the "Manual" mode and cook for 11 minutes at high pressure. Once cooking is complete, use a quick pressure release; carefully remove the lid. Transfer to wire racks.

Nutrition:

- Calories: 392 kcal
- Fat:18.7 g
- Carbohydrates: 50.1 g
- Protein: 5.9 g
- Sugar: 25.2 g
- Fiber: 0.7 g

130. Healthy Fruit Salad With Yogurt Cream

Preparation Time: 10 minutes

Cooking Time: 0 minutes

Servings: 4

Ingredients:

- 1½ cup grapes halved
- 2 plums, chopped
- 1 peach, chopped
- 1 cup cantaloupe, chopped
- ½ cup fresh blueberries
- 1 cup plain non-fat Greek yogurt, unsweetened
- ½ tsp cinnamon, ground
- 2 tbsp honey

Directions:

1. Mix the grapes, plums, peach, cantaloupe, and blueberries in a large bowl. Toss to mix. Divide among 4 dessert dishes.
2. In a small bowl, whisk the yogurt, cinnamon, and honey. Spoon over the fruit.
3. Sprinkle yogurt with sugar, and drizzle with honey. Serve fruit with a yogurt mixture.

Nutrition:

- Calories: 74 kcal
- Fat: 0.7 g
- Carbohydrates: 16 g
- Protein: 2 g

131. Summertime Fruit Salad

Cooking Time: 0 minutes

Preparation Time: 30 minutes

Servings: 6

Ingredients:

- 1-lb strawberries, hulled and sliced thinly
- 3 medium peaches, sliced thinly
- 6 oz blueberries
- 1 tbsp fresh mint, chopped
- 2 tbsp lemon juice
- 1 tbsp honey
- 2 tsp balsamic vinegar

Directions:

1. In a salad bowl, combine all ingredients.
2. Gently toss to coat all ingredients.
3. Chill for at least 30 minutes before serving.

Nutrition:

- Calories: 146 kcal
- Carbs: 22.8 g
- Protein: 8.1 g
- Fat: 3.4 g

132.   Popped Quinoa Bars

Preparation Time: 10 minutes

Cooking Time: 10 minutes

Servings: 3

Ingredients:

- 2 (4 oz) semi-sweet chocolate bars, chopped
- ½ tbsp peanut butter
- ½ cup dry quinoa
- ¼ tsp vanilla

Directions:

1. Toast dry quinoa in a pan until golden, and stir in chocolate, vanilla, and peanut butter.
2. Spread this mixture on a baking sheet evenly and refrigerate for about 4 hours.
3. Break it into small pieces and serve chilled.

Nutrition:

- Calories: 278 kcal
- Total Fat: 11.8 g
- Saturated Fat: 6.6 g
- Cholesterol: 7 mg
- Total Carbs: 36.2 g
- Dietary Fiber: 3.1 g
- Sugar: 15.4 g
- Protein: 6.9 g

133.   Almond Orange Pandoro

Preparation Time: 10 minutes

Cooking Time: 0 minutes

Servings: 12

Ingredients:

- 2 large oranges, zested
- 2½ cup mascarpone
- ½ cup almonds, whole
- 2½ cup coconut cream
- ½ pandoro, diced
- 2 tbsp sherry

Directions:

1. Whisk cream with mascarpone, icing sugar, ¾ zest, and half sherry in a bowl.
2. Dice the pandoro into equal-sized horizontal slices.
3. Place the bottom slice on a plate and top with the remaining sherry.
4. Spoon the mascarpone mixture over the slice.
5. Top with almonds and place another pandoro slice over.
6. Continue adding layers of pandoro slices and cream mixture. Dish out to serve.

Nutrition:

- Calories: 346 kcal
- Total Fat: 10.4 g
- Saturated Fat: 3 g
- Cholesterol: 10 mg
- Total Carbs: 8.5 g
- Dietary Fiber: 3 g
- Sugar: 2.4 g
- Protein: 7.7 g

134.   Blueberry Muffins

Preparation Time: 5 minutes

Cooking Time: 20 minutes

Servings: 24

Ingredients:

- 2 cups all-purpose flour
- 2 cups whole wheat flour
- ⅔ cup sugar

- 6 tsp baking powder
- 1 tsp salt
- 2 cups blueberries
- 2 free-range eggs
- ⅔ cup olive oil
- 2 cups milk

Directions:

1. Preheat your oven to 400°F and line a muffin tin with paper cases.
2. Grab a large bowl and add the dry ingredients. Stir well to combine.
3. Add the blueberries and stir through.
4. Take a medium bowl and add the wet ingredients. Stir well, then pour into the dry ingredients.
5. Pour the muffin batter into the muffin cases and pop it into the oven.
6. Bake for 18 minutes. Remove from the oven and allow to cool slightly before enjoying.

Nutrition:

- Calories: 179 kcal
- Net Carbs: 24 g
- Fat: 7 g
- Protein: 4 g

135. Mint Chocolate Chip Nice Cream

Preparation Time: 5 minutes

Cooking Time: -minutes

Servings: 1–2

Ingredients:

- 2 overripe bananas, frozen
- Pinch salt
- ⅛ tsp pure peppermint extract
- Pinch spirulina, or natural food coloring (optional)
- ½ cup coconut cream
- 2–3 tbsp chocolate chips

Directions:

1. Pop all the ingredients into your blender and whizz until smooth.
2. Serve and enjoy.

Nutrition:

- Calories: 601 kcal
- Net Carbs: 130 g
- Fat: 12 g
- Protein: 8 g

136. Creamy Berry Crunch

Preparation Time: 10 minutes

Cooking Time: 0 minutes

Servings: 2

Ingredients:

- 2 cups heavy cream for whipping
- 3 oz berries, fresh if possible
- The zest of half a lemon
- ¼ tsp vanilla extract
- 2 oz pecan nuts, chopped

Directions:

1. Into a large bowl, whip the cream until stiff.
2. Add the vanilla and the lemon zest and whip for a few seconds longer.
3. Add the nuts and the berries and stir in gently.
4. Place plastic cling film over the top of the bowl.
5. Serve!

Nutrition:

- Calories: 260 kcal
- Carbs: 3 g
- Fat: 27 g
- Protein: 3 g

137. Lemon Marmalade

Preparation Time: 10 minutes

Cooking Time: 15 minutes

Servings: 8

Ingredients:

- 2 lb lemons, washed, sliced, and cut into quarters
- 4 lb sugar
- 2 cups water

Directions:

1. Put the lemon pieces into the Instant Pot, add the water, cover, and cook on the Manual setting for 10 minutes.
2. Release the pressure naturally, uncover the Instant Pot, add the sugar, stir, set the Instant Pot on Manual mode, and cook for 6 minutes, stirring all the time.
3. Divide into jars, and serve when needed.

Nutrition:

- Calories: 100 kcal
- Fat: 2 g
- Fiber: 2 g
- Carbs: 4 g
- Protein: 8 g

138. Peach Jam

Preparation Time: 10 minutes

Cooking Time: 5 minutes

Servings: 6

Ingredients:

- 4½ cups peaches, peeled and cubed
- 6 cups sugar
- ¼ cup ginger, crystallized and chopped
- 1 box fruit pectin

Directions:

1. Set the Instant Pot on Manual mode, add the peaches, ginger, and pectin, stir, and bring to a boil.
2. Add the sugar, stir, cover, and cook on the Manual setting for 5 minutes.
3. Release the pressure, and uncover the Instant Pot.
4. Divide the jam into jars, and serve.

Nutrition:

- Calories: 50 kcal
- Fat: 0 g
- Fiber: 1 g
- Carbs: 3 g
- Protein: 0 g
- Sugar: 12 g

139. Greek-Style Compote With Yogurt

Preparation Time: 5 minutes

Cooking Time: 15 minutes

Servings: 4

Ingredients:

- 1 cup Greek yogurt
- 1 cup pears
- 4 tbsp honey
- 1 cup apples
- 1 vanilla bean
- 1 cinnamon stick
- ½ cup caster sugar
- 1 cup rhubarb
- 1 tsp ginger, ground
- 1 cup plums

Directions:

1. Place the fruits, ginger, vanilla, cinnamon, and caster sugar in the inner pot of the Instant Pot and secure the lid. Choose the Manual mode and cook for 2 minutes at high pressure. Once cooking is complete, use a natural pressure release for 10 minutes; carefully remove the lid. Meanwhile, whisk the yogurt with the honey.
2. Serve your compote in individual bowls with a dollop of honeyed Greek yogurt.

Nutrition:

- Calories: 304 kcal
- Fat: 0.3 g
- Carbohydrates: 75.4 g
- Protein: 5.1 g
- Sugar: 69.2 g

140. Butterscotch Lava Cakes

Preparation Time: 5 minutes

Cooking Time: 15 minutes

Servings: 6

Ingredients:

- 7 tbsp all-purpose flour
- A pinch coarse salt
- 6 oz butterscotch morsels

- ¾ cup sugar, powdered
- ½ tsp vanilla extract
- 3 eggs, whisked
- 1 stick butter

Directions:

1. Add 1 ½ cup water and a metal rack to the Instant Pot.
2. Line a standard-size muffin tin with muffin papers.
3. In a microwave-safe bowl, microwave butter and butterscotch morsels for about 40 seconds.
4. Stir in the powdered sugar.
5. Add the remaining ingredients.
6. Spoon the batter into the prepared muffin tin.
7. Secure the lid. Choose the Manual and cook at High pressure for 10 minutes. Once cooking is complete, use a quick release; carefully remove the lid.
8. To remove, let it cool for 5–6 minutes.
9. Run a small knife around the sides of each cake and serve.
10. Enjoy!

Nutrition:

- Calories: 393 kcal
- Fat: 21.1 g
- Carbohydrates: 45.6 g
- Protein: 5.6 g
- Sugar: 35.4 g

- 2 tbsp molasses
- 2 cups milk
- 4 cups Italian bread, cubed
- 1 tsp vanilla paste

Directions:

1. Add 1 ½ cup water and a metal rack to the Instant Pot.
2. Grease a baking dish with a nonstick cooking spray. Throw the bread cubes into the prepared baking dish.
3. In a mixing bowl, thoroughly combine the remaining ingredients. Pour the mixture over the bread cubes.
4. Cover with a piece of foil, making a foil sling.
5. Secure the lid. Choose the "Porridge" mode and high pressure; cook for 15 minutes.
6. Once cooking is complete, use a quick pressure release; carefully remove the lid.
7. Enjoy!

Nutrition:

- Calories: 410 kcal
- Fat: 24.3 g
- Carbohydrates: 37.4 g
- Protein: 11.5 g
- Sugar: 25.6 g

141. Vanilla Bread Pudding With Apricots

Preparation Time: 5 minutes

Cooking Time: 15 minutes

Servings: 6

Ingredients:

- 2 tbsp coconut oil
- 1⅓ cup heavy cream
- 4 eggs, whisked
- ½ cup apricots, dried, soaked, and chopped
- 1 tsp cinnamon, ground
- ½ tsp star anise, ground
- A pinch nutmeg, grated
- A pinch salt
- ½ cup sugar, granulated

Chapter 6. Bread Recipes

142. Fluffy Paleo Bread

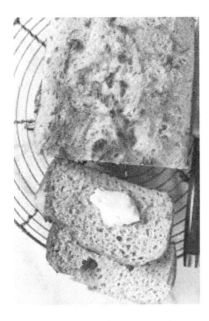

Preparation Time: 10 minutes

Cooking Time: 40 minutes

Servings: 15

Ingredients:

- 1¼ cup almond flour
- 5 eggs
- 1 tsp lemon juice
- ⅓ cup avocado oil
- 1 dash black pepper
- ½ tsp sea salt
- 3 to 4 tbsp tapioca flour
- 1 to 2 tsp poppy seed
- ¼ cup ground flaxseed
- ½ tsp baking soda
- Top with:
- Poppy seeds
- Pumpkin seeds

Directions:

1. Preheat the oven to 350°F.
2. Place the parchment paper on a baking sheet and set it aside.

3. In a bowl, add eggs, avocado oil, and lemon juice and whisk until combined.
4. Add tapioca flour, almond flour, baking soda, flaxseed, black pepper, and poppy seed to another bowl. Mix.
5. Add the lemon juice mixture into the flour mixture and mix well.
6. Add the batter into the prepared loaf pan and top with extra pumpkin seeds and poppy seeds.
7. Cover the loaf pan and transfer into the prepared oven.
8. Bake for 20 minutes. Remove cover and bake until an inserted knife comes out clean, after about 15–20 minutes.
9. Remove from oven and cool.
10. Slice and serve.

Nutrition:

- Calories: 149
- Fat: 12.9 g
- Carb: 4.4 g
- Protein: 5 g

143. Almond Bread

Preparation Time: 10 minutes

Cooking Time: 30 minutes

Servings: 20

Ingredients:

- 1½ cup almond flour
- 3 tsp baking powder
- 4 tbsp butter, melted
- ¼ tsp cream of tartar
- 6 eggs, whites and yolks separated
- Pinch of salt

Directions:

1. Preheat the oven to 375°F.
2. Grease a (8 x 4) inch loaf pan.
3. In a bowl, beat the cream of tartar and egg whites until soft peaks form.
4. Keep the mix on the side.
5. Mix the almond flour, salt, baking powder, egg yolks, and butter in a food processor.

6. Add ⅓ cups egg whites to the food processor and pulse until combined.
7. Add the rest of the egg whites and mix until combined.
8. Pour into the prepared loaf pan and bake for 30 minutes.
9. Cool, slice, and serve.

Nutrition:

- Calories: 271
- Fat: 22 g
- Carbs: 6 g
- Protein: 5 g

144. Iranian Flatbread

Preparation Time: 3 hours 15 minutes

Cooking Time: 6 minutes

Servings: 6

Ingredients:

- 4 cups almond flour
- 2½ cups warm water
- 1 tbsp instant yeast
- 12 tsp sesame seeds
- Salt to taste

Directions:

1. In a bowl, add 1 tbsp yeast to ½ cup warm water. Let stand for 5 minutes to activate. Add salt and 1 cup of water. Let stand for 10 minutes more.
2. Add flour 1 cup at a time, and then add the remaining water.
3. Knead the dough, shape it into a ball, and let stand for 3 hours covered.
4. Preheat the oven to 480°F.
5. With a rolling pin, roll out the dough and divide it into 6 balls. Roll each ball into ½-inch thick rounds.
6. Line a baking sheet with parchment paper and place the rolled rounds on it. Make a small hole in the middle with a finger and add 2 tsp sesame seeds to each hole. Bake for 3–4 minutes and then flip over and bake for 2 minutes more.

Nutrition:

- Calories: 26
- Fat: 1 g
- Carbs: 3.5 g
- Protein: 1 g

145. Double Chocolate Zucchini Bread

Preparation Time: 10 minutes

Cooking Time: 55 minutes

Servings: 12

Ingredients:

- ½ cup coconut flour
- ½ cup chocolate chips (sugar-free)
- 2 cups zucchini (shredded)
- 1 tsp vanilla
- 4 large eggs
- ¼ cup coconut oil, melted
- ¼ tsp salt
- 1 tsp baking powder
- 1 tsp baking soda
- ½ tsp ground cinnamon
- ½ cup low-carb sweetener
- ½ cup cocoa powder (unsweetened)

Directions:

1. In a bowl, combine coconut flour, salt, baking powder, cinnamon, sweetener, baking soda, and cocoa.
2. Blend in the vanilla, coconut oil, and eggs.
3. Mix well.
   Fold in the chocolate chips and zucchini.
4. Line a loaf pan (9 x 5) with parchment paper and pour the mixture into it.
5. Bake at 350°F for 45–55 minutes.
6. Remove from the oven and cool.
7. Serve and enjoy!

Nutrition:

- Calories: 124
- Fat: 10 g
- Carbs: 7 g
- Protein: 4 g

146. Bread De Soul

Preparation Time: 10 minutes

Cooking Time: 45 minutes

Servings: 16

Ingredients:

- ¼ tsp cream of tartar
- 2½ tsp baking powder
- 1 tsp xanthan gum
- ⅓ tsp baking soda
- ½ tsp salt
- 1 ⅔ cup unflavored whey protein
- ¼ cup olive oil
- ¼ cup heavy whipping cream or half and half
- 2 drops of sweet leaf stevia
- 4 eggs
- ¼ cup butter
- 12 oz softened cream cheese

Directions:

1. Preheat the oven to 325°F.
2. In a bowl, microwave cream cheese and butter for 1 minute.
3. Remove and blend well with a hand mixer.
4. Add olive oil, eggs, heavy cream, and a few drops of sweetener and blend well.
5. Blend the dry ingredients in a clean bowl.
6. Combine the dry ingredients with the wet ingredients and mix with a spoon. Don't use a hand blender to avoid whipping it too much.
7. Grease a bread pan and pour the mixture into the pan.
8. Bake in the oven until golden brown, about 45 minutes.
9. Cool and serve.

Nutrition:

- Calories: 200
- Fat: 15.2 g
- Carbs: 1.8 g
- Protein: 10 g

147. Sesame Bread

Preparation Time: 5 minutes

Cooking Time: 30 minutes

Servings: 8

Ingredients:

- 1 cup almond flour
- 7 oz cream cheese
- 4 eggs
- 4 tbsp sesame oil
- 1 tsp salt
- 2 tbsp ground psyllium husk powder
- 1 tbsp sesame seeds
- 1 tsp baking powder
- Sea salt

Directions:

1. Preheat the oven to 400°F.
2. Whisk the eggs until a fluffy consistency is reached.
3. Add cream cheese and sesame oil to the beaten egg and mix well.
4. Add every other ingredient into the mixture, excluding the sesame seeds, and stir unit mixed.
5. Pour dough into a parchment paper-lined baking sheet.
6. Let sit for 5 minutes and cover dough top with sesame oil.
7. Sprinkle the dough with salt and sesame seeds.
8. Bake for 30 minutes, or until the top is golden and well cooked.
9. Cool, slice, and serve.

Nutrition:

- Calories: 282
- Fat: 26 g
- Carbs: 2 g
- Protein: 7 g

148. Cauliflower Bread Loaf

Preparation Time: 1 hour 10 minutes

Cooking Time: 45 minutes

Servings: 10

Ingredients:

For the Bread Dough:

- 1¼ cup of almond flour
- 3 cups of riced cauliflower
- 1 tbsp baking powder

- 6 tbsp of olive oil
- 6 large eggs, separated
- 1 tsp salt

Optional Flavorings:

- Dried or fresh herbs
- Shredded parmesan or cheddar cheese
- Garlic powder or minced garlic

Directions:

1. Preheat the oven to 350°F. Line a bread loaf with baking paper.
2. Place cauliflower into the small pot to steam until it becomes tender. Place it to the side.
3. Cream the whites of the eggs in a food processor for 4 minutes. Set to the side.
4. In a bowl, whisk the egg yolks and almond flour until mixed well. Next, add the baking powder, oil, and salt and mix until smooth.
5. Remove excess fluid from the cooled cauliflower with a paper towel.
6. Stir in the dried cauliflower and mix well. Add the flavoring ingredients.
7. In small amounts, fold the egg white mixture into the mixture until fluffy. Don't overbeat.
8. Transfer the dough into the bread loaf pan.
9. Bake in the oven for 45 minutes. Test with a knife.
10. Cool, slice, and serve.

Nutrition:

- Calories: 155
- Fat: 13 g
- Carbs: 4 g
- Protein: 3 g

149. Cloud Bread Cheese

Preparation Time: 5 minutes

Cooking Time: 30 minutes

Servings: 12

Ingredients:

For Cream Cheese Filling:

- 1 egg yolk
- ½ tsp vanilla stevia drops for filling
- 8 oz softened cream cheese

Base Egg Dough:

- ½ tsp cream of tartar
- 1 tbsp coconut flour
- ¼ cup unflavored whey protein
- 3 oz softened cream cheese
- ¼ tsp vanilla stevia drops for dough
- 4 eggs, separated

Directions:

1. Preheat the oven to 325°F.
2. Line 2 baking sheets with parchment paper.
3. In a bowl, stir the 8 oz of cream cheese, stevia, and egg yolk.
4. Transfer to the pastry bag.
5. In another bowl, separate egg yolks from whites.
6. Add 3 oz cream cheese, yolks, stevia, whey protein, and coconut flour. Mix until smooth.
7. Whip cream of tartar with the egg whites until stiff peaks form.
8. Fold the yolk/cream cheese mixture into the beaten whites.
9. Spoon batter onto each baking sheet, 6 mounds on each. Press each mound to flatten a bit.
10. Add cream cheese filling in the middle of each batter.
11. Bake for 30 minutes at 325°F.

Nutrition:

- Calories: 120
- Fat: 10.7 g
- Carbs: 1.1 g
- Protein: 5.4 g

150. Cinnamon Swirl Almond Bread

Preparation Time: 15 minutes

Cooking Time: 40 minutes

Servings: 16

Ingredients:

- 2½ cups almond flour
- ¼ cup chopped walnuts
- ¼ cup melted coconut oil
- 4 eggs
- ½ cup hot water
- ½ cup erythritol

- 1 tbsp cinnamon + 2 tsp
- ½ tsp salt
- 1 tsp baking powder
- 4 tbsp psyllium husk

Directions:

1. Preheat the oven to 375°F.
2. Mix erythritol, 1 tbsp cinnamon, salt, baking powder, psyllium husk, and almond flour in a bowl.
3. Add hot water and mix well.
4. Add coconut oil and eggs and mix.
5. Grease an 8-inch bread pan and pour half the batter.
6. Sprinkle 2 tsp of cinnamon on top.
7. Pour the remaining batter into the pan.
8. Make a swirl with a knife.
9. Sprinkle with chopped walnuts.
10. Bake in the oven for 40 minutes.
11. Serve.

Nutrition:

- Calories: 166
- Fat: 14 g
- Carbs: 7 g
- Protein: 5 g

151. Lime Blueberry Bread

Preparation Time: 15 minutes

Cooking Time: 35 minutes

Servings: 16

Ingredients:

- 3 cups almond flour, blanched
- 2 tbsp egg white protein powder
- ½ tsp baking soda
- 1 tsp cream of tartar
- 6 large eggs
- ¼ tsp sea salt
- ½ tsp vanilla stevia
- 1 tbsp lime zest
- 1 cup frozen blueberries

Directions:

1. Preheat the oven to 350°F and grease a loaf pan.
2. Add almond flour, protein powder, cream of tartar, baking soda, and salt to a food processor.
3. Pulse mixture to combine.
4. Mix and add stevia, eggs, and lime zest into the food processor and pulse until you get a very smooth batter.
5. Add blueberries into the batter and stir until mixed.
6. Pour batter into the prepared loaf pan and transfer to the preheated oven.
7. Bake for 45–55 minutes, and cool for 2 hours.
8. Slice and serve.

Nutrition:

- Calories: 231
- Fat: 18 g
- Carbs: 8 g
- Protein: 12 g

152. Chia Seed Bread

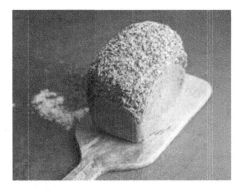

Preparation Time: 10 minutes

Cooking Time: 40 minutes

Servings: 16 slices

Ingredients:

- ½ tsp xanthan gum
- ½ cup butter
- 2 tbsp coconut oil
- 1 tbsp baking powder
- 3 tbsp sesame seeds
- 2 tbsp chia seeds
- ½ tsp salt
- ¼ cup sunflower seeds
- 2 cups almond flour
- 7 eggs

Directions:

1. Preheat the oven to 350°F.
2. Beat eggs in a clean bowl on high for 1–2 minutes.
3. Beat in the xanthan gum and combine coconut oil and melted butter into eggs, beating continuously.
4. Set aside the sesame seeds, but add the rest of the ingredients.
5. Line a loaf pan with baking paper and place the mixture in it. Top the mixture with sesame seeds.
6. Bake in the oven until a toothpick inserted comes out clean, about 35–40 minutes.

Nutrition:

- Calories: 405
- Fat: 37 g
- Carbs: 4 g
- Protein: 14 g

153. Splendid Low-Carb Bread

Preparation Time: 15 minutes

Cooking Time: 60–70 minutes

Servings: 12

Ingredients:

- ½ tsp herbs, such as basil, rosemary, or oregano
- ½ tsp garlic or onion powder
- 1 tbsp baking powder
- 5 tbsp psyllium husk powder
- ½ cup almond flour
- ½ cup coconut flour
- ¼ tsp salt
- 1½ cup egg whites
- 3 tbsp oil or melted butter
- 2 tbsp apple cider vinegar
- ⅓ to ¾ cup hot water

Directions:

1. Grease a loaf pan and preheat the oven to 350°F.
2. Whisk the salt, psyllium husk powder, onion or garlic powder, coconut flour, almond flour, and baking powder in a bowl.

3. Stir in egg whites, oil, and apple cider vinegar. Bit by bit, add the hot water, stirring until the dough increase in size. Do not add too much water.
4. Mold the dough into a rectangle and transfer to a grease loaf pan.
5. Bake in the oven for 60–70 minutes or until the crust feels firm and brown on top.
6. Cool and serve.

Nutrition:

- Calories: 97
- Fat: 5.7 g
- Carbs: 7.5 g
- Protein: 4.1 g

154. Coconut Flour Almond Bread

Preparation Time: 10 minutes

Cooking Time: 30 minutes

Servings: 4

Ingredients:

- 1 tbsp butter, melted
- 1 tbsp coconut oil, melted
- 6 eggs
- 1 tsp Baking soda
- 2 tbsp ground flaxseed
- 1½ tbsp psyllium husk powder
- 5 tbsp coconut flour
- 1½ cup almond flour

Directions:

1. Preheat the oven to 400°F. Mix the eggs in a bowl for a few minutes.
2. Add in the butter and coconut oil and mix once more for 1 minute.
3. Add the almond flour, coconut flour, baking soda, psyllium husk, and ground flaxseed to the mixture. Let sit for 15 minutes.
4. Lightly grease the loaf pan with coconut oil. Pour the mixture into the pan.
5. Place in the oven and bake until a toothpick inserted in it comes out dry about 25 minutes.

Nutrition:

- Calories: 475
- Fat: 38 g
- Carbs: 7 g
- Protein: 19 g

155. Quick Low-Carb Bread Loaf

Preparation Time: 45 minutes

Cooking Time: 40–45 minutes

Servings: 16

Ingredients:

- ⅔ cup coconut flour
- ½ cup butter, melted
- 3 tbsp coconut oil, melted
- 1⅓ cup almond flour
- ½ tsp xanthan gum
- 1 tsp baking powder
- 6 large eggs
- ½ tsp salt

Directions:

1. Preheat the oven to 350°F. Cover the bread loaf pan with baking paper.
2. Beat the eggs until creamy.
3. Add in the coconut flour and almond flour, mixing them for 1 minute. Next, mix the xanthan gum, coconut oil, baking powder, butter, and salt until the dough becomes thick.
4. Put the completed dough into the prepared line of the bread loaf pan.
5. Place in oven and bake for 40–45 minutes. Check with a knife. Slice and serve.

Nutrition:

- Calories: 174
- Fat: 15 g
- Carbs: 5 g
- Protein: 5 g

156. Cheese Garlic Bread

Preparation Time: 10 minutes

Cooking Time: 15 minutes

Servings: 10

Ingredients:

- 170 g mozzarella cheese, shredded
- 85 g almond meal
- 1 tbsp crushed garlic
- 2 tbsp full-fat cream cheese
- 1 tsp baking powder
- 1 tbsp dried parsley
- 1 medium egg
- 1 pinch salt

Directions:

1. Add every ingredient into a bowl, excluding the egg. Stir the mixture until combined.
2. Place bowl in a microwave and microwave for 1 minute on high.
3. Stir the mixture and microwave for 30 seconds more.
4. Add the egg into the dough and gently stir until incorporated.
5. Add mixture onto a prepared baking tray and mold into a loaf shape.
6. Sprinkle any leftover cheese over the bread.
7. Bake loaf for 15 minutes at 425°F or until golden brown.

Nutrition:

- Calories: 117.4
- Fat: 9.8 g
- Carbs: 2.4 g
- Protein: 6.2 g

157. Almond Flour Lemon Bread

Preparation Time: 15 minutes

Cooking Time: 45 minutes

Servings: 16

Ingredients:

- 1 tsp French herbs
- 1 tsp lemon juice
- 1 tsp salt
- 1 tsp cream of tartar
- 2 tsp baking powder
- ¼ cup melted butter
- 5 large eggs, divided
- ¼ cup coconut flour
- 1½ cup almond flour

Directions:

1. Preheat the oven to 350°F.
2. Whip the whites and cream of tartar until soft peaks form.
3. Combine salt, egg yolks, melted butter, and lemon juice in a bowl. Mix well.
4. Add coconut flour, almond flour, herbs, and baking powder. Mix well.
5. To the dough, add ⅓ the egg whites and mix until well-combined.
6. Add the remaining egg whites mixture and slowly mix to incorporate everything. Do not over mix.
7. Grease a loaf pan with butter or coconut oil.
8. Pour mixture into the loaf pan and bake for 30 minutes.
9. Serve and enjoy!

Nutrition:

- Calories: 115
- Fat: 9.9 g
- Carbs: 3.3 g
- Protein: 5.2 g

158. Seed and Nut Bread

Preparation Time: 10 minutes

Cooking Time: 40 minutes

Servings: 24

Ingredients:

- 3 eggs
- ¼ cup avocado oil
- 1 tsp psyllium husk powder
- 1 tsp apple cider vinegar
- ¾ tsp salt
- 5 drops liquid stevia
- 1½ cup raw unsalted almonds
- ½ cup raw unsalted pepitas
- ½ cup raw unsalted sunflower seeds
- ½ cup flaxseeds

Directions:

1. Preheat the oven to 325°F. Line a loaf pan with parchment paper.

2. Whisk together the oil, eggs, psyllium husk powder, vinegar, salt, and liquid stevia in a large bowl. Stir in the pepitas, almonds, sunflower seeds, and flaxseeds.
3. Pour the batter into the prepared loaf pan, smooth it out and let it rest for 2 minutes.
4. Bake for 40 minutes. Cool, slice, and serve.

Nutrition:

- Calories: 131
- Fat: 12 g
- Carbs: 4 g
- Protein: 5 g

159. Blueberry Bread Loaf

Preparation Time: 20 minutes

Cooking Time: 65 minutes

Servings: 12

Ingredients:

For the Bread Dough:

- 10 tbsp coconut flour
- 9 tbsp melted butter
- ⅔ cup granulates swerve sweetener
- 1½ tsp baking powder
- 2 tbsp heavy whipping cream
- 1½ tsp vanilla extract
- ½ tsp cinnamon
- 2 tbsp sour cream
- 6 large eggs
- ½ tsp salt
- ¾ cup blueberries

For the Topping:

- 1 tbsp heavy whipping cream
- 2 tbsp confectioner swerve sweetener
- 1 tsp melted butter
- ⅛ tsp vanilla extract
- ¼ tsp lemon zest

Directions:

1. Preheat the oven to 350°F and line a loaf pan with baking paper.
2. Mix granulated swerve, heavy whipping cream, eggs, and baking powder in a bowl.

3. Once combined, add the butter, vanilla extract, salt, cinnamon, and sour cream. Then add the coconut flour to the batter.
4. Pour a layer of about ½ inch of dough into the bread pan. Place ¼ cup of blueberries on top of the dough. Keep repeating until the dough and blueberry layers are complete.
5. Bake for 65–75 minutes.
6. Meanwhile, in a bowl, beat the vanilla extract, butter, heavy whipping cream, lemon zest, and confectioner swerve. Mix until creamy.
7. Cool the bread once baked. Then drizzle the icing topping on the bread.
8. Slice and serve.

Nutrition:

- Calories: 155
- Fat: 13 g
- Carbs: 4 g
- Protein: 3 g

160.   Herbed Garlic Bread

Preparation Time: 10 minutes

Cooking Time: 45 minutes

Servings: 10

Ingredients:

- ½ cup coconut flour
- 8 tbsp melted butter, cooled
- 1 tsp baking powder
- 6 large eggs
- 1 tsp garlic powder
- 2 tsp rosemary, dried
- ¼ tsp salt
- ½ tsp onion powder

Directions:

1. Add coconut flour, baking powder, onion, garlic, rosemary, and salt into a bowl. Combine and mix well. Add the eggs into another bowl and beat until bubbly on top. Add melted butter
2. Add bacon and jalapeño mix. Grease the loaf pan with ghee. Pour batter into the loaf pan and bake for 40 mins. Serve and enjoy.

Nutrition:

into the bowl with the eggs and beat until mixed.
2. Gradually add the coconut flour mixture to the egg mixture.
3. Mix with a hand mixer. Preheat the oven to 350°F and prepare a greased loaf pan.
4. Pour batter into the prepared loaf pan and even the top with a spatula.
5. Transfer the loaf pan to the preheated oven and bake for 40–50 mins. Cool and slice.

Nutrition:

- Calories: 147
- Fat: 12.5 g
- Carbs: 3.5 g
- Protein: 4.6 g

161.   Spicy Bread

Preparation Time: 10 minutes

Cooking Time: 40 minutes

Servings: 6

Ingredients:

- ½ cup coconut flour
- 6 eggs
- 3 large jalapeños, sliced
- 4 oz turkey bacon, sliced
- ½ cup ghee
- ¼ tsp baking soda
- ¼ tsp salt
- ¼ cup water

Directions: Preheat the oven to 400°F. Cut bacon and jalapenos on a baking tray and roast for 10 minutes. Flip and bake for 5 more minutes. Remove seeds from the jalapeños. Place jalapeños and bacon slices in a food processor and blend until smooth. In a bowl, add ghee, eggs, and ¼-cup water. Mix well.

1. Then add the coconut flour, baking soda, and salt. Stir to mix.

Calories: 240

- Fat: 20 g
- Carb: 5 g
- Protein: 9 g

Chapter 7. Side Dish Recipes

162.   Moroccan Style Couscous

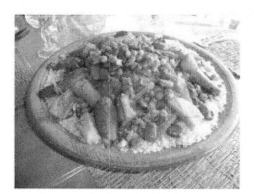

Preparation Time: 10 minutes

Cooking Time: 10 minutes

Servings: 4

Ingredients:

- 1 cup yellow couscous
- ½ tsp ground cardamom
- 1 cup chicken stock
- 1 tbsp butter
- 1 tsp salt
- ½ tsp red pepper

Directions:

1. Set butter in the pan and melt it. Attach couscous and roast it for 1 minute over high heat. Then, add ground cardamom, salt, and red pepper.
2. Stir it well. Pour the chicken stock and bring the mixture to a boil.
3. Set and simmer couscous for 5 minutes with a closed lid.

Nutrition:

- Calories: 196
- Fat: 3.4 g
- Fiber: 2.4 g
- Carbs: 35 g
- Protein: 5.9 g

163.   Creamy Polenta

Preparation Time: 8 minutes

Cooking Time: 45 minutes

Servings: 4

Ingredients:

- 1 cup polenta
- 1½ cup water
- 2 cups chicken stock
- ½ cup cream
- ⅓ cup Parmesan, grated

Directions:

1. Put polenta in the pot. Add water, chicken stock, cream, and Parmesan.
2. Mix up polenta well. Then preheat the oven to 355°F.
3. Cook polenta in the oven. Merge up the cooked meal with the help of the spoon carefully before serving.

Nutrition:

- Calories: 208
- Fat: 5.3 g
- Fiber: 1 g
- Carbs: 32.2
- Protein: 8 g

164.   Mushroom Millet

Preparation Time: 10 minutes

Cooking Time: 15 minutes

Servings: 3

Ingredients:

- ¼ cup mushrooms, sliced
- ¾ cup onion, diced
- 1 tbsp olive oil
- 1 tsp salt
- 3 tbsp milk
- ½ cup millet
- 1 cup of water
- 1 tsp butter

Directions:

1. Set olive oil in the skillet, then put the onion. Attach mushrooms and roast the vegetables for 10 minutes over medium heat. Stir them from time to time.
2. Meanwhile, pour water into the pan. Add millet and salt. Cook the millet with the closed lid over medium heat.
3. Then, add the cooked mushroom mixture to the millet, the milk and butter. Mix up the millet well.

Nutrition:

- Calories: 198
- Fat: 7.7 g
- Fiber: 3.5 g
- Carbs: 27.9 g
- Protein: 4.7 g

165. Spicy Barley

Preparation Time: 7 minutes

Cooking Time: 42 minutes

Servings: 5

Ingredients:

- 1 cup barley
- 3 cups chicken stock
- ½ tsp cayenne pepper
- 1 tsp salt
- ½ tsp chili pepper
- ½ tsp ground black pepper
- 1 tsp butter
- 1 tsp olive oil

Directions:

1. Set barley and olive oil in the pan. Roast barley on high heat.
2. Stir well. Then add the salt, chili, ground black pepper, cayenne pepper, and butter, followed by the chicken stock.
3. Secure the lid and cook barley for 40 minutes over medium-low heat.

Nutrition:

- Calories: 152
- Fat: 2.9 g

- Fiber: 6.5 g
- Carbs: 27.8 g
- Protein: 5.1 g

166. Tender Farro

Preparation Time: 8 minutes

Cooking Time: 40 minutes

Servings: 4

Ingredients:

- 1 cup farro
- 3 cups beef broth
- 1 tsp salt
- 1 tbsp almond butter
- 1 tbsp dried dill

Directions:

1. Set farro in the pan. Add beef broth, dried dill, and salt.
2. Secure the lid and place the mixture to boil. Then boil it for 35 minutes over medium-low heat. When finished, open the lid, and add almond butter.
3. Mix up the cooked farro well.

Nutrition:

- Calories: 95
- Fat: 3.3 g
- Fiber: 1.3 g
- Carbs: 10.1 g
- Protein: 6.4 g

167. Wheat Berry Salad

Preparation Time: 10 minutes

Cooking Time: 50 minutes

Servings: 2

Ingredients:

- ¼ cup of wheat berries
- 1 cup of water
- 1 tsp salt
- 2 tbsp walnuts, chopped
- 1 tbsp chives, chopped

- ¼ cup fresh parsley, chopped
- 2 oz pomegranate seeds
- 1 tbsp canola oil
- 1 tsp chili flakes

Directions:

1. Set wheat berries and water in the pan. Attach salt and simmer the ingredients for 50 minutes over medium heat.
2. Meanwhile, merge together walnuts, chives, parsley, pomegranate seeds, and chili flakes. When the wheat berry is cooked, put it in the walnut mixture.
3. Attach canola oil and mix up the salad well.

Nutrition:

- Calories: 160
- Fat: 11.8 g
- Fiber: 1.2 g
- Carbs: 12 g
- Protein: 3.4 g

168. Curry Wheat Berry Rice

Preparation Time: 10 minutes

Cooking Time: 1 hour 15 minutes

Servings: 5

Ingredients:

- 1 tbsp curry paste
- ¼ cup milk
- 1 cup wheat berries
- ½ cup of rice
- 1 tsp salt
- 4 tablespoons olive oil
- 6 cups chicken stock

Directions:

1. Place the wheat berries and chicken stock in the pan. Secure the lid and cook the mixture for 1 hour over medium heat. Then add rice, olive oil, and salt.
2. Stir well. Mix up together milk and curry paste. Attach the curry liquid to the rice-wheat berry mixture and stir well. Set the meal for 15 minutes with a closed lid.

3. When the rice is processed, all the meal is cooked.

Nutrition:

- Calories: 232
- Fat: 15 g
- Fiber: 1.4 g
- Carbs: 23.5 g
- Protein: 3.9 g

169. Couscous Salad

Preparation Time: 10 minutes

Cooking Time: 6 minutes

Servings: 4

Ingredients:

- ⅓ cup couscous
- ⅓ cup chicken stock
- ¼ tsp ground black pepper
- ¾ tsp ground coriander
- ½ tsp salt
- ¼ tsp paprika
- ¼ tsp turmeric
- 1 tbsp butter
- 2 oz chickpeas, canned, drained
- 1 cup fresh arugula, chopped
- 2 oz sun-dried tomatoes, chopped
- 1 oz Feta cheese, crumbled
- 1 tbsp canola oil

Directions:

1. Bring the chicken stock to a boil.
2. Add couscous, black pepper, coriander, salt, paprika, and turmeric. Attach chickpeas and butter.
3. Set the mixture well and close the lid.
4. Meanwhile, combine arugula, sun-dried tomatoes, and Feta cheese in the bowl.
5. Add cooked couscous mixture and canola oil.
6. Mix up the salad well.

Nutrition:

- Calories: 18
- Fat: 9 g
- Fiber: 3.6 g
- Carbs: 21.1 g

- Protein: 6 g

170. Farro Salad With Arugula

Preparation Time: 10 minutes

Cooking Time: 35 minutes

Servings: 2

Ingredients:

- ½ cup farro
- 1½ cup chicken stock
- 1 tsp salt
- ½ tsp ground black pepper
- 2 cups arugula, chopped
- 1 cucumber, chopped
- 1 tbsp lemon juice
- ½ tsp olive oil
- ½ tsp Italian seasoning

Directions:

1. Merge together farro, salt, and chicken stock and transfer the mixture to the pan. Secure the lid and boil it for 35 minutes.
2. Meanwhile, set all remaining ingredients in the salad bowl. Chill the farro and add it to the salad bowl too.
3. Mix up the salad well.

Nutrition:

- Calories: 92
- Fat: 2.3 g
- Fiber: 2 g
- Carbs: 15.6 g
- Protein: 3.9 g

171. Cauliflower Broccoli Mash

Preparation Time: 5 minutes

Cooking Time: 10 minutes

Servings: 6

Ingredients:

- 1 large head cauliflower, cut into chunks
- 1 small head broccoli, cut into florets
- 3 tablespoons extra virgin olive oil

- 1 tsp salt
- Pepper, to taste

Directions:

1. Set a pot and add oil, then heat it. Add the cauliflower and broccoli. Flavor with salt and pepper to taste. Keep stirring.
2. Add water if needed. When it is already cooked, puree the vegetables using a food processor or a potato masher.
3. Serve and enjoy!

Nutrition:

- Calories: 39
- Fat: 3 g
- Carbohydrates: 2 g
- Protein: 0.89 g

172. Broccoli & Black Beans Stir Fry

Preparation Time: 10 minutes

Cooking Time: 15 minutes

Servings: 4

Ingredients:

- 4 cups broccoli florets
- 1 tbsp sesame oil
- 4 tsp sesame seeds
- 2 tsp ginger, finely chopped
- A pinch turmeric powder
- Lime juice to taste (optional)
- 2 cups cooked black beans
- 2 cloves garlic, finely minced
- A large pinch red chili flakes
- Salt to taste

Directions:

1. Set enough water to cover the bottom of the saucepan by an inch.
2. Place a strainer on the saucepan.
3. Place broccoli florets on the strainer.
4. Steam the broccoli for 6 minutes.
5. Set a large frying pan over medium heat.
6. Add sesame oil.
7. When the oil is warm, add the sesame seeds, chili flakes, ginger, garlic, turmeric powder, and salt. Sauté.

8. Add steamed broccoli and black beans and sauté until thoroughly heated.
9. Add lime juice and stir.
10. Serve hot.

Nutrition:

- Calories: 196 kcal
- Protein: 11.2 g
- Fat: 7.25 g
- Carbohydrates: 23.45 g

173. Roasted Curried Cauliflower

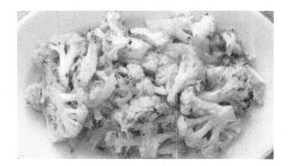

Preparation Time: 5 minutes

Cooking Time: 30 minutes

Servings: 4

Ingredients:

- 1 large head cauliflower, cut into florets
- 1 tsp curry powder
- 1 ½ tbsp olive oil
- 1 tsp cumin seeds
- 1 tsp mustard seeds
- ¾ tsp salt

Directions:

1. Preheat your oven to 375°F.
2. Grease a baking sheet with cooking spray.
3. Take a bowl and place all ingredients.
4. Toss to coat well.
5. Arrange the vegetable on a baking sheet.
6. Roast for 30 minutes.
7. Serve and enjoy!

Nutrition:

- Calories: 67
- Fat: 6 g

- Carbs: 4 g
- Protein: 2 g

174. Caramelized Pears & Onions

Preparation Time: 5 minutes

Cooking Time: 35 minutes

Servings: 4

Ingredients:

- 2 red onions, cut into wedges
- 2 firm red pears, cored and quartered
- 1 tbsp olive oil
- Salt and pepper, to taste

Directions:

1. Preheat your oven to 425°F.
2. Set the pears and onion on a baking tray.
3. Drizzle with olive oil.
4. Season with salt and pepper.
5. Bake in the oven for 35 minutes.
6. Serve and enjoy!

Nutrition:

- Calories: 101
- Fat: 4 g
- Carbs: 17 g
- Protein: 1 g

175. Cool Garbanzo & Spinach Beans

Preparation Time: 5–10 minutes

Cooking Time: 5 minutes

Servings: 4

Ingredients:

- 12 oz garbanzo beans
- 1 tbsp olive oil
- ½ onion, diced
- ½ tsp cumin
- 10 oz spinach, chopped

Directions:

1. Set a skillet and add olive oil.
2. Set it over medium-low heat.

3. Attach onions and garbanzo, and cook for 5 minutes.
4. Set in cumin, garbanzo beans, spinach, and season with sunflower seeds.
5. Use a spoon to smash gently.
6. Cook thoroughly.
7. Serve and enjoy!

Nutrition:

- Calories: 90
- Fat: 4 g
- Carbs: 11 g
- Protein: 4 g

176. Onion & Orange Healthy Salad

Preparation Time: 10 minutes

Cooking Time: 0 minutes

Servings: 3

Ingredients:

- 6 large oranges
- 3 tbsp Red wine vinegar
- 6 tbsp olive oil
- 1 tsp oregano, dried
- 1 red onion, thinly sliced
- 1 cup black olives
- ¼ cup fresh chives, chopped
- Ground black pepper

Directions:

1. Set the orange and cut each of them into 4–5 crosswise slices.
2. Set the oranges on a shallow dish.
3. Whisk the vinegar and olive oil, sprinkle the oregano, and toss.
4. Set sliced onion and black olives on top.
5. Serve and enjoy!

Nutrition:

- Calories: 120
- Fat: 6 g
- Carbs: 20 g
- Protein: 2 g

177. Olive & Tomato Balls

Preparation Time: 10 minutes

Cooking Time: 35 minutes

Servings: 5

Ingredients:

- 5 tbsp parmesan cheese, grated
- ¼ tsp salt
- Black pepper (as desired)
- 2 garlic cloves, crushed
- 4 Kalamata olives, pitted
- 4 pcs sun-dried tomatoes, drained
- 2 tbsp oregano, chopped
- 2 tbsp Thyme, chopped
- 2 tbsp basil, chopped
- ¼ cup coconut oil
- ½ cup cream cheese

Directions:

1. Slice the coconut oil, add it to a small mixing bowl with the cream cheese, and leave them to soften for about 30 minutes.
2. Smash together and mix well to combine.
3. Attach in the Kalamata olives and sun-dried tomatoes and mix well before adding in the herbs and seasonings.
4. Merge thoroughly before placing the mixing bowl in the refrigerator to allow the results to solidify.
5. Once it has solidified, set the mixture into a total of 5 balls using an ice cream scoop.
6. Set each of the finished balls into the parmesan cheese before plating.
7. Store the extra's in the fridge in an air-tight container for up to 7 days.

Nutrition:

- Calories: 212
- Protein: 4.77 g
- Fat: 20.75 g
- Carbs: 3.13 g

178. Apple & Berries Ambrosia

Preparation Time: 15 minutes

Cooking Time: 0 minutes

Servings: 4

Ingredients:

- 2 cups unsweetened coconut milk, chilled
- 2 tbsp raw honey
- 1 apple, peeled, cored, and chopped
- 2 cups fresh raspberries
- 2 cups fresh blueberries

Directions:

1. Set the chilled milk in a large bowl, then mix in the honey. Stir to mix well.
2. Then add and mix the remaining ingredients.
3. Stir to coat the fruits well and serve them immediately.

Nutrition:

- Calories: 386
- Fat: 21.1 g
- Protein: 4.2 g
- Carbs: 45.9 g

179.   Banana, Cranberry & Oat Bars

Preparation Time: 15 minutes

Cooking Time: 40 minutes

Servings: 16 bars

Ingredients:

- 2 tbsp extra-virgin olive oil
- 2 medium ripe bananas, mashed
- ½ cup almond butter
- ½ cup maple syrup
- ⅓ cup dried cranberries
- 1½ cup old-fashioned rolled oats
- ¼ cup oat flour
- ¼ cup ground flaxseed
- ¼ tsp ground cloves
- ½ cup shredded coconut
- ½ tsp ground cinnamon
- 1 tsp vanilla extract

Directions:

1. Preheat the oven to 400°F (205°C).
2. Set an 8-inch square pan with parchment paper, then grease with olive oil.

3. Combine the mashed bananas, almond butter, and maple syrup in a bowl. Stir to mix well.
4. Merge in the remaining ingredients and stir to mix well until thick and sticky.
5. Spread the mixture evenly on the square pan with a spatula, then bake for 40 minutes or until a toothpick inserted in the center comes out clean.
6. Remove them from the oven and slice them into 16 bars to serve.

Nutrition:

- Calories: 145
- Fat: 7.2 g
- Protein: 3.1 g
- Carbs: 18.9 g

180.   Berry and Rhubarb Cobbler

Preparation Time: 15 minutes

Cooking Time: 35 minutes

Servings: 8

Ingredients:

Cobbler:

- 1 cup fresh raspberries
- 2 cups fresh blueberries
- 1 cup sliced (½-inch) rhubarb pieces
- 1 tbsp arrowroot powder
- ¼ cup unsweetened apple juice
- 2 tbsp melted coconut oil
- ¼ cup raw honey

Topping:

- 1 cup almond flour
- 1 tbsp arrowroot powder
- ½ cup shredded coconut
- ¼ cup raw honey
- ½ cup coconut oil

Directions:

1. Preheat the oven to 350°F (180c). Set a baking dish with melted coconut oil. Combine the ingredients for the cobbler in a large bowl. Stir to mix well. Spread the mixture in a single layer on the baking dish. Set aside.

2. Combine the almond flour, arrowroot powder, and coconut in a bowl. Stir to mix well. Fold in the honey and coconut oil. Stir with a fork until the mixture crumbled.
3. Spread the topping over the cobbler, then bake in the preheated oven for 35 minutes or until bubbly and golden brown. Serve immediately.

Nutrition:

- Calories: 305
- Fat: 22.1 g
- Protein: 3.2 g
- Carbs: 29.8 g

181. Citrus Cranberry & Quinoa Energy Bites

Preparation Time: 15 minutes

Cooking Time: 0 minutes

Servings: 12 bites

Ingredients:

- 2 tbsp almond butter
- 2 tbsp maple syrup
- ¾ cup cooked quinoa
- 1 tbsp dried cranberries
- 1 tbsp chia seeds
- ¼ cup ground almonds
- ¼ cup sesame seeds, toasted
- Zest of 1 orange
- ½ tsp vanilla extract

Directions:

1. Line a baking sheet with parchment paper. Merge the butter and maple syrup in a bowl. Stir to mix well.
2. Fold in the remaining ingredients and stir until the mixture holds together and is smooth. Set the mixture into 12 equal parts, then shape each part into a ball.
3. Arrange the balls on the baking sheet, then refrigerate for at least 15 minutes. Serve chilled.

Nutrition:

- Calories: 110
- Fat: 10.8 g
- Protein: 3.1 g

- Carbs: 4.9 g

182. Chocolate, Almond & Cherry Clusters

Preparation Time: 15 minutes

Cooking Time: 3 minutes

Servings: 10 clusters

Ingredients:

- 1 cup dark chocolate (60% cocoa or higher), chopped
- 1 tbsp coconut oil
- ½ cup dried cherries
- 1 cup roasted salted almonds

Directions:

1. Line a baking sheet with parchment paper. Dissolve the chocolate and coconut oil in a saucepan for 3 minutes. Stir constantly.
2. Turn off the heat and mix in the cherries and almonds. Drop the mixture on the baking sheet with a spoon. Place the sheet in the refrigerator and chill for at least 1 hour or until firm. Serve chilled.

Nutrition:

- Calories: 197
- Fat: 13.2 g
- Protein: 4.1 g
- Carbs: 17.8 g

183. Chocolate & Avocado Mousse

Preparation Time: 15 minutes

Cooking Time: 5 minutes

Servings: 4–6

Ingredients:

- 8 oz (227 g) dark chocolate (60% cocoa or higher), chopped
- ¼ cup unsweetened coconut milk
- 2 tbsp coconut oil
- 2 ripe avocados, deseeded
- ¼ cup raw honey

- Sea salt, to taste

Directions:

1. Put the chocolate in a saucepan. Set in the coconut milk and add the coconut oil. Cook for 3 minutes or until the chocolate and coconut oil melt. Stir constantly.
2. Put the avocado in a food processor, then drizzle with honey and melted chocolate. Pulse to combine until smooth.
3. Pour the mixture into a serving bowl, then sprinkle with salt. Refrigerate to chill for 30 minutes and serve.

Nutrition:

- Calories: 654
- Fat: 46.8 g
- Protein: 7.2 g
- Carbs: 55.9 g

184. Coconut Blueberries With Brown Rice

Preparation Time: 15 minutes

Cooking Time: 10 minutes

Servings: 4

Ingredients:

- 1 cup fresh blueberries
- 2 cups unsweetened coconut milk
- 1 tsp ground ginger
- ¼ cup maple syrup
- Sea salt, to taste
- 2 cups cooked brown rice

Directions:

1. Put all the ingredients, except for the brown rice, in a pot. Stir to combine well. Cook until the blueberries are tender.
2. Pour in the brown rice and cook for 3 more minutes or until the rice is soft. Stir constantly. Serve immediately.

Nutrition:

- Calories: 470
- Fat: 24.8 g
- Protein: 6.2 g
- Carbs: 60.1 g

Chapter 8. Vegan and Vegetarian Recipes

- Sodium: 148 mg

185. Broccoli-Sesame Stir-Fry

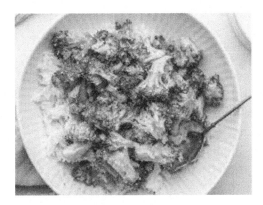

Preparation Time: 10 minutes

Cooking Time: 10 minutes

Servings: 4

Ingredients:

- 2 tbsp extra-virgin olive oil
- 1 tsp sesame oil
- 4 cups broccoli florets
- 1 tbsp grated fresh ginger
- ¼ tsp sea salt
- 2 garlic cloves, minced
- 2 tbsp toasted sesame seeds

Directions:

1. Heat the olive oil and sesame oil in a large non-stick skillet over medium-high heat until they shimmer.
2. Add the broccoli, ginger, and salt.
3. Add the garlic. Cook for 30 seconds, stirring constantly.
4. Remove from the heat and stir in the sesame seeds.

Nutrition:

- Calories: 134
- Fat: 11 g
- Protein: 4 g
- Carbs: 9 g
- Fiber: 3 g
- Sugar: 2 g

186. Whitefish Curry

Preparation Time: 15 minutes

Cooking Time: 15 minutes

Servings: 4–6

Ingredients:

- 2 tbsp coconut oil
- 1 onion, chopped
- 2 garlic cloves, minced
- 1 tbsp minced fresh ginger
- 2 tsp curry powder
- 1 tsp salt
- ¼ tsp freshly ground black pepper
- 1 (4-inch) piece lemongrass (white part only), bruised with the back of a knife
- 2 cups cubed butternut squash
- 2 cups chopped broccoli
- 1 (13½-oz / 383-g) can coconut milk
- 1 cup vegetable broth, or chicken broth
- 1 pound (454 g) firm whitefish fillets
- ¼ cup chopped fresh cilantro
- 1 scallion, sliced thinly
- Lemon wedges, for garnish

Directions:

1. In a large pot over medium-high heat, melt the coconut oil. Add the onion, garlic, ginger, curry powder, salt, and pepper.
2. Sauté for 5 minutes.
3. Add the lemongrass, butternut squash, and broccoli. Sauté for 2 minutes more.
4. Stir in the coconut milk and vegetable broth and bring to a boil. Reduce the heat to simmer and add the fish. Cover the pot and simmer for 5 minutes, or until the fish is cooked through. Remove and discard the lemongrass.
5. Ladle the curry into a serving bowl. Garnish with the cilantro and scallion, and serve with the lemon wedges.

Nutrition:

- Calories: 553

- Fat: 39 g
- Protein: 34 g
- Carbs: 22 g
- Fiber: 6 g
- Sugar: 7 g
- Sodium: 881 mg

187. Braised Bok Choy With Shiitake Mushrooms

Preparation Time: 10 minutes

Cooking Time: 10 minutes

Servings: 4

Ingredients:

- 1 tbsp coconut oil
- 8 baby bok choy, halved lengthwise
- ½ cup water
- 1 tbsp coconut aminos
- 1 cup shiitake mushrooms, stemmed, sliced thinly
- Salt, to taste
- Freshly ground black pepper, to taste
- 1 scallion, sliced thinly
- 1 tbsp toasted sesame seeds

Directions:

1. In a large pan over high heat, melt the coconut oil. Add the bok choy in a single layer.
2. Add the water, coconut aminos, and mushrooms to the pan. Cover and braise the vegetables for 5–10 minutes or until the bok choy is tender.
3. Remove the pan from the heat. Season the vegetables with salt and pepper.
4. Transfer the bok choy and mushrooms to a serving dish and garnish with the scallions and sesame seeds.

Nutrition:

- Calories: 285
- Fat: 8 g
- Protein: 26 g
- Carbs: 43 g
- Fiber: 18 g
- Sugar: 21 g
- Sodium: 1035 mg

188. Rich in Nutrients Noodles With Tahini and Kale

Preparation Time: 5 minutes

Cooking Time: 8–10 minutes

Servings: 4

Ingredients:

- 8 oz brown rice spaghetti or buckwheat noodles
- 4 cups kale, lightly packed
- ½ cup tahini
- ¾ cup hot water, plus additional as needed
- ¼ tsp salt, plus additional as needed
- ½ cup fresh parsley, chopped

Directions:

1. Cook the noodles according to the package Directions.
2. Toss in the kale during the last 30 seconds of cook time. Drain the noodles and kale in a colander. Transfer to a large bowl.
3. Stir together the tahini, hot water, and salt in a medium bowl. Add more water if you prefer a thinner sauce. Add the parsley and sauce to the noodles. Toss to coat. Taste and adjust the seasoning if necessary. Serve hot or cold.

Nutrition:

- Calories: 404
- Fat: 18 g
- Carbs: 54 g
- Sugar: 2 g
- Fiber: 10 g
- Protein: 15 g
- Sodium: 223 mg

189. Lentil & Quinoa Salad

Preparation Time: 5 minutes

Cooking Time: 15 minutes

Servings: 4

Ingredients:

- 2 medium green apples, cored, chopped
- 3 cups cooked quinoa

- ½ of a medium red onion, peeled, diced
- 3 cups cooked green lentils
- 1 large carrot, shredded
- 1 ½ tsp salt
- 1 tsp ground black pepper
- 2 tbsp olive oil
- ¼ cup balsamic vinegar

Directions:

1. Take a large bowl, place all the ingredients, and then stir until combined.
2. Let the salad chill in the refrigerator for 1 hour, divide it evenly among 6 bowls, and then serve.

Nutrition:

- Calories: 199 Cal
- Fat: 10.7 g
- Protein: 8 g
- Carbs: 34.8 g
- Fiber: 5.9 g

190. Potato Salad

Preparation Time: 5 minutes

Cooking Time: 25 minutes

Servings: 4

Ingredients:

- 2 medium potatoes
- 2 medium tomatoes, diced
- 2 celery, diced
- 1 green onion, chopped

Directions:

1. Place the potatoes into a pan, cover with water, and then place the pan over medium-high heat.
2. Cook the potatoes for 20 minutes, and when done, drain them and let them cool.
3. Peel the potatoes cut them into cubes, and then place them into a large bowl.
4. Add tomatoes, celery, and green onion, season with salt and black pepper, drizzle with oil and then toss until coated.
5. Divide the salad between 3 bowls and then serve.

Nutrition:

- Calories: 268.5
- Fat: 15.8 g
- Protein: 5 g
- Carbs: 21 g
- Fiber: 2.5 g

191. Zucchini Pepper Chips

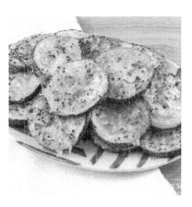

Preparation Time: 10 minutes.

Cooking Time: 15 minutes.

Servings: 4

Ingredients:

- 1⅔ cup vegetable oil
- 1 tsp onion powder
- ½ tsp black pepper
- 3 tbsp red pepper flakes, crushed
- 2 zucchinis, thinly sliced

Directions:

1. Mix oil with all the spices in a bowl.
2. Add zucchini slices and mix well.
3. Transfer the mixture to a Ziplock bag and seal it.
4. Refrigerate for 10 minutes.
5. Spread the zucchini slices on a greased baking sheet.
6. Bake for 15 minutes
7. Serve.

Nutrition:

- Calories: 172 kcal
- Fat: 11.1 g
- Carbs: 19.9 g
- Protein: 13.5 g

192.   Super Seed Spelt Pancakes

Preparation Time: 15 minutes

Cooking Time: 10 minutes

Servings: 3

Ingredients:

- 5 oz buckwheat groats
- 1½ tsp cinnamon, ground
- 1½ oz flax seeds
- 1½ oz sesame seeds
- 2 oz chia seeds
- 1 oz pumpkin seeds
- 1 tbsp almond milk
- ½ tsp stevia extract
- 1 tsp coconut oil
- 1 tsp baking soda
- ½ tsp baking powder
- ¼ tsp fine sea salt

Directions:

1. Grind the pumpkin seeds, sesame seeds, flax seeds, chia seeds, and buckwheat groats into flour and keep ¼ of the seed flour for later use (not for this recipe).
2. Add 2 cups of seed flour to a medium bowl.
3. Add in the rest of the ingredients but not the coconut oil.
4. Pour in more milk if needed to attain the right consistency.
5. Once heated, pour thin layers of the batter and flip once you see bubbles form on top.
6. Cook until all the batter is used up.

Nutrition:

- Calories: 140 kcal
- Fiber: 12 g
- Protein: 34 g

193.   Scrambled Tofu

Preparation Time: 10 minutes

Cooking Time: 15 minutes

Servings: 1

Ingredients:

- 3 cloves
- 1 onion
- ½ tsp turmeric
- Salt for taste
- 2 oz firm tofu
- ½ tsp paprika
- 1 handful baby spinach
- 3 tomatoes
- ½ cup yeast
- ½ tsp cumin

Directions:

1. Mince the garlic and dice up the onion.
2. Toss the onions into a pan and let them cook over medium heat for about 7 minutes.
3. Toss in the tofu and tomatoes and cook for 10 more minutes. Add in some water, cumin, and paprika, and stir well. Continue cooking.
4. When the dish is about to cook, add in spinach, stir, and once wilted, turn off the heat and serve.

Nutrition:

- Calories: 151 kcal
- Protein: 29 g
- Fat:10 g

194.   Tofu Salad

Preparation Time: 10 minutes

Cooking Time: 15 minutes

Servings: 2

Ingredients:

- ½ pack firm tofu
- ½ a red onion
- 2 spelled tortillas
- 1 avocado
- 4 handfuls baby spinach
- 1 handful almonds
- 2 tomatoes
- 1 pink grapefruit
- ½ lemon

Directions:

1. Heat the tortillas in an oven, and bake for 8–10 minutes in the oven.

2. Chop up the onions, tomatoes, and tofu and combine this. Put it in the fridge and let it cool.
3. Now chop up the almonds, avocado, and grapefruit. Mix everything well and place nicely around the bowl you had put in the fridge.
4. Squeeze a lemon on top all over the salad, and enjoy!

Nutrition:

- Calories: 110 kcal
- Fiber: 12 g
- Protein: 36 g

195. Tofu & Tomato

Preparation Time: 15 minutes

Cooking Time: 15 minutes

Servings: 2

Ingredients:

- 1 tbsp coconut oil
- A little coriander/cilantro
- 10 oz regular firm tofu
- 2 large handfuls of baby spinach
- ½ brown onion (or red if you fancy)
- 1 handful arugula/rocket
- Black pepper, freshly ground
- 2 tomatoes
- Himalayan/Sea salt
- Pinch turmeric
- A little basil
- ½ small red pepper
- A pinch cayenne pepper

Directions:

1. Use your hands to scramble the tofu into a bowl, then chop and fry the onion quickly in a pan. Dice the peppers and do the same thing.
2. Dice the tomatoes and throw them into the pan. Toss in a pinch of turmeric, and add the spinach. Add salt and grind in the pepper. Cook until the tofu is warm and cooked.
3. Throw in basil leaves, coriander, the rocket just when the meal is about to be done. Serve with a pinch of some hot cayenne pepper.
4. You can serve on some toasted sprouted bread and some baby spinach.

Nutrition:

- Calories: 174 kcal
- Fiber: 10 g
- Protein: 27 g

196. Lentil-Stuffed Potato Cakes

Preparation Time: 15 minutes

Cooking Time: 30 minutes

Servings: 4

Ingredients:

For the Cakes:

- Salt
- 1 bay leaf
- 10 medium gold potatoes
- 1 cup potato starch- add more for dusting

For the Stuffing:

- Coconut oil for pan-frying
- Salt and black pepper, freshly ground
- 1 medium onion, chopped
- 4 oz mushrooms
- 2 tbsp olive oil
- ¾ cup green lentils, dried and cooked (preferably French lentils)

Directions:

1. Combine the 7 cups of water, potatoes, and bay leaf in a large pot and boil until the potatoes are tender. Poke with a fork to ensure they are cooked.
2. Rinse the potatoes under cold water when done; the skins will peel off easily. Now mash the potatoes until smooth and add the potato starch; stir to make the dough. Add more potato starch if the dough feels too sticky.
3. For the stuffing, add olive oil to a sauté pan and place over medium-high heat. Add in onions and cook as you stir for 5 minutes. Add in the lentils with pepper and salt (to taste) and cook for 2 minutes. Set aside.
4. To make the cakes, scoop about 3 tbsp of the dough on your hand and press it into your palm.
5. Add a spoonful of stuffing on top of the dough and fold it over to close it. Shape it into a round disk.

6. Now add coconut oil to a skillet and heat over medium heat. Cook the potato cakes on both sides until golden, roughly 4 minutes per side.

Nutrition:

- Calories: 227 kcal
- Fat:1 g
- Protein: 41 g

197. Sesame Ginger Cauliflower Rice

Preparation Time: 10 minutes

Cooking Time: 15 minutes

Servings: 4

Ingredients:

- 2 tbsp wheat-free tamari plus more to taste
- 4 cups mushrooms, finely chopped
- 1 large head cauliflower
- 2 tbsp sesame oil, toasted
- 2 tbsp grapeseed oil
- ½ tsp Celtic Sea salt, plus more to taste
- 6 green onions, finely chopped (white and green parts)
- 1 bunch cilantro, finely chopped (½ C.)
- 2 tbsp fresh ginger, minced
- 2 tsp fresh lime juice, plus more to taste
- 1 small green chili, ribbed, seeded, and minced
- 4 tsp garlic cloves, minced

Directions:

1. For the cauliflower rice, roughly cut the cauliflower into florets and get rid of the tough middle core.
2. Fit a food processor with an S blade and add the florets to pulse. Pulse for a few seconds until the florets achieve a rice-like consistency. You should have 5–6 cups of rice in the end.
3. Heat oil in a deep skillet or wok over medium-high heat and fry the ginger, green onions, chili, garlic, and mushroom seasoned with ¼ tsp of salt for 5 minutes. Once combined well and soft, add in the tamari and cauliflower rice and cook for 5 more minutes until soft.
4. Add in the remaining salt, cilantro, and lime juice, and adjust the flavors as desired.
5. Serve and enjoy!

Nutrition:

- Calories: 113 kcal
- Fiber: 14 g
- Fat:7 g

198. Spinach With Chickpeas & Lemon

Preparation Time: 10 minutes

Cooking Time: 15 minutes

Servings: 2

Ingredients:

- 3 tbsp extra virgin olive oil
- Sea salt, to taste (i.e., Celtic Grey, Himalayan, or Redmond Real Salt)
- ½ container grape tomatoes
- 1 large can chickpeas, rinse well
- 1 large onion, thinly sliced
- 1 tbsp ginger, grated
- 1 large lemon, zested and freshly juiced
- 1 tsp red pepper flakes, crushed
- 4 garlic cloves, minced

Directions:

1. Pour the olive oil into a large skillet and add the onion. Cook for about 5 minutes until the onion starts to brown.
2. Add in the ginger, lemon zest, garlic, tomatoes, and red pepper flakes and cook for 3–4 minutes.
3. Toss in the chickpeas (rinsed and drained) and cook for an additional 3–4 minutes. Now add the spinach in 2 batches, and once it starts to wilt, season with some sea salt and lemon juice.
4. Cook for 2 minutes.

Nutrition:

- Calories: 239 kcal
- Protein: 28 g
- Fat:5 g

199. Kale Wraps With Chili & Green Beans

Preparation Time: 30 minutes

Cooking Time: 0 minute

Servings: 2

Ingredients:

- 1 tbsp fresh lime juice
- 1 tbsp raw seed mix
- 2 large kale leaves
- 2 tsp fresh garlic, finely chopped
- ½ ripe avocado, pitted and sliced
- 1 tsp fresh red chili, seeded and finely chopped
- 1 cup fresh cucumber sticks
- Fresh coriander leaves, finely chopped
- 1 cup green beans

Directions:

1. Spread kale leaves on a clean kitchen work surface.
2. Spread each chopped coriander leaves on each leaf, position them around the end of the leaf, perpendicular to the edge.
3. Spread green beans equally on each leaf, at the edge of each leaf, the same as the coriander leaves.
4. Do the same thing with the cucumber sticks.
5. Cut the divided chopped garlic across each leaf, sprinkling it all over the green beans.
6. Cut and share the chopped chili across each leaf and sprinkle it over the garlic.
7. Now, divide the avocado across each leaf, and spread it over chili, garlic, coriander, and green beans.
8. Share the raw seed mix among each leaf, and sprinkle them over other ingredients.
9. Divide the lime juice across each leaf and drizzle it over all other ingredients.
10. Now fold or roll up the kale leaves and wrap up all the ingredients within them.
11. You can serve it with soy sauce!

Nutrition:

- Calories: 328 kcal
- Fiber: 12 g
- Protein: 42 g

200. Cabbage Wraps With Avocado & Strawberries

Preparation Time: 30 minutes

Cooking Time: 0 minutes

Servings: 1–2

Ingredients:

- ½ cup raw pecan nuts, roughly chopped
- ½ cup fresh strawberries, sliced
- 2 large cabbage leaves
- ½ ripe avocado
- 1 cup green asparagus spears

Directions:

1. Spread out the cabbage sheets on a clean kitchen work surface.
2. Share the asparagus shear among each cabbage leaf and place them on the edge of the leaf.
3. Share the avocado slices on each leaf and put them on top of the asparagus spears.
4. Share the strawberries over each leaf and spread them on top of the avocado slices.
5. Share the pecan nuts between each leaf and spread them on the strawberries.
6. Wrap the leaves with all ingredients inside them.
7. Serve with soy sauce (optional).

Nutrition:

- Calories: 176 kcal
- Protein: 34 g
- Fiber: 11 g

Chapter 9. 28-day Meal Plan

Below is a 28-day meal plan to help you get started with the anti-inflammatory diet. Combining all the recipes in this cookbook can make a 1900-day meal plan.

Days	Breakfast	Lunch/dinner	Dessert/snack
1	Mexican breakfast toast	Chicken bone broth	Vanilla ice cream
2	Italian breakfast hash	Chicken bone broth with ginger and lemon	Rich carob sheet cake
3	Papaya breakfast boat	Vegetable stock	Banana "nice" cream
4	Summer medley parfait	Chicken vegetable soup	Key lime pie pots de crème
5	Banana pancakes	Carrot ginger soup	Apricot biscotti
6	Mango salsa	Turkey sweet potato hash	Chocolate mascarpone
7	Avocado gazpacho	Turkey taco lettuce boats	Almond ricotta spread
8	Mango banana smoothie	Turkey and greens meatloaf	Baklava with lemon honey syrup
9	Toxin flush smoothie	Simple italian seasoned turkey breast	Greek butter cookies
10	Berry peach smoothie	Spiced chicken and vegetables	Cocoa muffins with coffee

11	Veggie avocado smoothie	Lemon garlic turkey breast	Low carb nougat whims
12	Apple blueberry smoothie	Home-style chicken and vegetables	Raspberry feast meringue with cream diplomat
13	Alkaline papaya smoothie	Greek baked cod	Cheesecake mousse with raspberries
14	Heart-healthy berry smoothie	Pork and chestnuts mix	Almond meringue cookies
15	Watermelon smoothie	Chicken and butter sauce	Maple-glazed pears with hazelnuts
16	Lettuce and orange smoothie	Chicken tacos	Gluten-free oat and fruit bars
17	Detox apple smoothie	Turkey verde with brown rice	Banana cherry smoothie
18	Berries and hemp seeds smoothie	Greek chicken bites	Blueberry and spinach smoothie
19	Pear, berries, and quinoa smoothie	Lemon chicken	Matcha mango smoothie
20	Chia seed pudding	Chicken shawarma	Pecan and lime cheesecake
21	Scrambled eggs	Lemon chicken mix	Roasted potatoes

22	Muesli-style oatmeal	Balsamic chicken	Pumpkin zucchini muffins
23	Steel cut oatmeal	Chicken and olives salsa	White bean basil hummus
24	Breakfast porridge	Seafood noodles	Garlic rosemary roasted nuts
25	Mushroom omelet with bell pepper	Tuna bowl with kale	Recipe for ruby pears delight
26	Scrambled eggs with smoked salmon	Tuna with vegetable mix	Mixed berry and orange compote
27	Scotch eggs with ground turkey	Paprika butter shrimps	Fig and homey buckwheat pudding
28	Green berry smoothie	Garlic and shrimp pasta	Zingy blueberry sauce

To receive your FREE eBook "The 8 Week Shred" Scan this QR Code

Chapter 10. Ten Simple Physical Exercises Suitable for Everyone to Start and Get Fit and Achieve the Goals You Want in Just 21 Days

Burpees

The burpee is a push-up variation that works multiple muscles at once. To perform a burpee, begin with a push-up and immediately roll onto your back, bending your legs and attempting to touch your elbows to the floor. After one push-up, you jump up and perform as many burpees as you can in a row before lowering yourself to the ground. If you can do 15 push-ups, you should be able to do 10 burpees in a row (you can always keep going after reaching the number of burpees you set out to complete).

Crab Crawl

Similar to a burpee, the crab crawl works a variety of muscles and is just as difficult. To do this exercise, start by lying on your back and then kick your legs into the air so that you are in sit-up position. Raise your bottom off the ground (until your feet reach 90 degrees), then lower yourself down to the ground for 10 seconds before repeating this movement a total of 30 times.

Jumping Jacks

It is an excellent exercise for anyone who enjoys dancing or doing aerobics because it works several different muscles at the same time. To do jumping jacks, simply stand up straight and jump as high as you can in the air while bringing your arms together above your head and then back to your sides after touching your feet.

Crunches

To do a crunch, lie on the floor face up with your head resting on a mat (or towel) and with hands placed behind your head. Then bring knees to the chest while raising shoulders and upper body off the ground. Make sure you hold that position for 5 seconds before slowly returning to the original position.

Donkey Kick

The donkey kick is a great upper body exercise that also works the abdominal muscles. Hold on to a chair for support and balance, then wrap a towel around your feet and lift your bottom off the ground by bending only at the knees. Then, while keeping the rest of your body still, bring your legs up in a straight position (as if you were trying to put your head between them). When you finish one donkey kick, slowly lower yourself to the ground before rising again.

Walking Lunges

A variation on lunges where instead of using weights (or no equipment at all) you walk forward with hands stretched above your head, alternating legs after each step. To do this exercise, start by standing with feet apart for balance and then step forward about 6–8 feet with your left leg. Now extend your left leg behind you and keep your toes pointing forward. After that, step forward with your right leg and bring your arms back down to the starting position. Repeat this movement on the opposite side.

Abdominal Sit-ups

The abdominal sit-up, also known as a "crunch," is a good exercise for strengthening the abdominal muscles. Begin an abdominal sit-up by lying face up on the floor, legs straight in the air, and hands behind the head. You might only be able to reach halfway up at first. After that, you should be able to completely lift your torso off the floor with straight legs (and bring it back down slowly).

Side Plank

The side plank is a fantastic way to work both sides of your abs simultaneously and strengthen your shoulders. To do this exercise, start by lying on your side on the ground and then lift one knee upwards while keeping the other leg bent and resting on the floor. Make sure that your shoulder blades touch either side of your buttocks when you breathe out hard (exhale normally).

Squats

Squats, another exercise that works many muscles at once, are excellent for strengthening multiple muscle groups and increasing lower-body flexibility. To perform a squat, first, stand with your feet apart for balance, then squat as far as you can with your knees in line with your feet. Return to your starting position and repeat the movement while keeping your knees relatively high (but not lower than the hips).

Sailing

This fantastic exercise combines a lot of different movements in one exercise, so it is ideal for working those muscles that are difficult to reach, such as belly muscles. To do this exercise, get into the push-up position, then start by lifting your arms out to the side while keeping your head up straight. Then bring hands together and raise the body off the ground while moving arms in an outwardly rotating circular motion. After that, return to the original position slowly before lowering yourself down again.

Conclusion

Thank you for reading this book. Many people suffer from inflammation, a common ailment characterized by symptoms such as pain, redness, and swelling. Inflammation is also a reaction to injury or rejection of the body's own tissues. To help reduce the effects of inflammation, avoid activities that cause it and, if necessary, take a cocktail of anti-inflammatory drugs.

Inflammation is not only painful, but it can also lead to serious complications like diabetes and heart disease in people who are unable to control it with medication alone. Inflammation can be caused by a variety of factors, including poor diet, injuries, stress, certain medications, and cigarette smoking.

It is critical to pay close attention to any signs your body may send you and not become discouraged if you do not see results immediately. However, it can take a long time for the body to heal itself and restore balance naturally.

It is also important to remember that many different factors can contribute to inflammation in the body, and that these can vary from person to person (ex: stress, depression, anxiety). This is why it is critical for you as an individual to pay close attention to your own body by taking regular measurements so that you know what works and what does not.

The most important thing is to listen to your body rather than your mind. Finally, keep in mind that there are numerous factors that can cause inflammation in the body, and it is critical to monitor any changes in your daily routine. If you notice any significant changes, you may require the assistance of someone with more experience with natural remedies to improve your health.

Thank you for getting this far. I have spent so much time writing this manuscript, and now I kindly ask you to help me with the popularization. This would mean so much to me; it would really give me immense pleasure to receive a positive review from you on Amazon; your reviews are much more important than you know!

Index

Made in the USA
Las Vegas, NV
24 January 2023

66214137R00057